Advance Praise for *Save Your Mind*

"With advice that is actionable, in language that is sharp, Dr. Hakim shows, explains, and sensitizes. As he uncovers the human dimensions of the disease and what can be done, he enables us to care better for ourselves, and others. This book is a gift, an invitation to the human spirit, a call to our formidable capacity to engage in combat and change course. Armed with love, determination, empathy, and the very memories that are under attack, everyone can take steps today so the future doesn't take away the present, then the past. This book is for everyone who owns a brain."

— Michaëlle Jean, Secretary General of La Francophonie and Governor General of Canada (2005 to 2010)

"Dr. Hakim's book shines a light on the critical importance of brain health: what we put in our heads helps protect us from both stroke and dementia. The book emphasizes the brain's constant need for good blood supply, and describes how vascular risk factors such as high blood pressure can be managed through long-term regular physical activity, healthy eating, good sleep habits, avoiding loneliness, and exercising the brain by learning new activities. This book raises awareness around the risk of dementia and provides essential and practical information for anyone who wishes to reduce the risk for this awful condition."

— Dr. Patrice Lindsay, Director, Stroke, Heart & Stroke Foundation

"Dementia is a huge problem, and this impressive book can help each one of us reduce our risk for it."

— Dr. Yves Joanette, Chair, World Dementia Council

"When approaching middle or old age, who of us has not been afraid of the possibility of developing dementia? In a well-researched book, Dr. Hakim outlines seven practical measures each of us can take to prevent, or at least postpone, this unpleasant disease."

— François Mai, MD, FRCPC, FRCP (Ed), Adjunct Professor, Faculty of Medicine, Queen's University, and author of Diagnosing Genius: The Life and Death of Beethoven

SAVE YOUR MIND

Seven Rules to Avoid Dementia

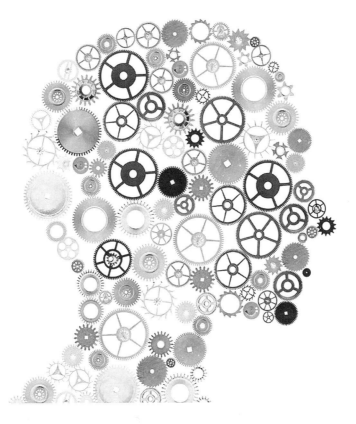

Antoine Hakim, O.C., MD, PhD, FRCPC

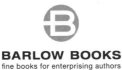

BARLOW BOOKS
fine books for enterprising authors

Library and Archives Canada Cataloguing in Publication data available upon request.

ISBN 978-1-988025-21-6

Printed in Canada

In Canada:
Georgetown Publications
34 Armstrong Avenue, Georgetown, ON L7G 49R

In the U.S.A.:
Midpoint Book Sales & Distribution
27 West 20th Street, Suite 1102, New York, NY 10011

For more information, visit **www.barlowbooks.com**

Barlow Book Publishing Inc.
96 Elm Avenue, Toronto, ON
Canada M4W 1P2

BARLOW BOOKS

For my grandmother and parents, who despite forced migrations and extreme poverty remained committed to their children's success and happiness.

For my wife and children, who lovingly understood and accepted my prolonged commitment to writing this book.

Contents

List of Figures

List of Tables

Introduction

Why You Need to Read This Book . . . and Follow Its Seven Rules

This book will help you keep your marbles!

We are all getting older, we're living longer, and we're terrified of losing our minds and having dementia. This book is written because I believe I have advice that will substantially reduce your likelihood of having dementia. The main lesson my 40 years of neurology practice have taught me is that vascular disease affecting the brain, combined with harmful behavioural patterns, contributed to dementia in the majority of cases. This combination usually led to sufficient damage to the brain's structure and integrity that normal thinking and memory recall became difficult if not impossible.

This book is not intended only for the older citizen. It is now clear that the script for dementia is written very early, perhaps as early as our teenage years, so this book is written for everyone who cares about keeping the mind healthy. In my neurology practice, I have seen patients in their 40s who complained of "brain fog" and were clearly staring at the abyss of dementia. Some were able to reverse course and avoid that outcome while others continued their downhill path and over a few years became heavily dependent on their environment.

In the following pages, I will share with you knowledge I have gained from research done in Canada, the United States, and internationally on the topic of strokes and other vascular diseases that affect the brain. I will advise you especially on how to avoid them. I will also share with you knowledge on how to acquire some patterns of behaviour and avoid others in order to preserve your cognitive abilities. Lectures I have given internationally on the topic were always so popular that I decided to include in this book advice on how to maintain your ability to think and remember. You will learn how memory works in our brains and how to distinguish normal forgetfulness from more sinister possibilities.

The important message in this book is this: *The risk of dementia is modifiable.*

We do not have to acquire dementia as we age. There are lots of good examples of individuals, and even entire societies, where people remain intellectually sharp into very old age. I will give several examples of healthy minds in old age and extract from the accumulated studies advice you need to follow to stay sharp. To accomplish this, I have summarized current knowledge into seven rules to guide your future mental and cognitive health. These seven rules are based on my clinical experience, published research work, and voracious reading of the medical literature. The rules will benefit every person interested in preserving their mind and their ability to think and remember.

So read, enjoy, and get with the program.

Happy reading!

Before the Rules,
A Few Facts

We Are Living Longer, But We Also Want Good Life Quality

Dementia is by and large a disease that accompanies old age, and all of us are hoping, indeed expecting, that we will live longer than our parents did. Statistics confirm this expectation of longevity. They tell us that currently 50 million Americans are older than 65, and that in Canada 16% of the population is in that category. This demographic group is growing faster than any other. Not only that, but the rate of growth of this group is accelerating. Once Americans reach the age of 65, the average remaining life expectancy is still 20.4 years for women and 17.8 years for men.

It's not just that we are living longer; our attitude towards old age is also changing. I saw an obituary recently that said, "Jo Smith died unexpectedly at the age of 93." While we are of course delighted that life's joys may be ours for longer than we anticipated, our fervent desire is not just to live long in years. We also want good life quality. And for most of us that means keeping our marbles and our independence as we age. We are aware deep in our souls that without the health of our brain and our mind, there is no health.

The statistics about life quality are daunting. Currently it is estimated, using different calculation methods, that more than 500,000 Canadians, 5 million U.S. citizens, and 44 million individuals worldwide suffer from dementia.[1] If you include individuals affected by milder forms of memory difficulty, not severe enough to qualify for dementia, these figures grow by about 50%. As if that was not bad enough, it is also estimated that every five minutes, one person somewhere is diagnosed with dementia.

And of course, those individuals afflicted with dementia are not the only ones affected by the condition. Every person with dementia requires a caregiver, frequently a family member whose chances of becoming depressed increase dramatically over time. Usually, both the affected individual and the care provider need to quit work, stop deriving income, and stop paying taxes. For this reason, there is increasing concern that what some refer to as the "dementia time bomb" will result in a severe fiscal squeeze: spending on age-related programs, including health care for seniors, will have to increase at a time when declining birth rates will result in diminishing revenues. This will force governments to increase taxes and modify health care systems to give priority to this debilitating condition, taking funding away from other projects and health care needs.

David Cameron, the former prime minister of the United Kingdom, called dementia one of the "greatest enemies of humanity." Against this unsettling background, there is good news, and that is why this book was written.

Let me start with a story from my own family. My father-in-law is 91 years old. He fought in the Second World War as an Air Corps gunner, and when he returned home he worked as a carpenter. He has always been physically active. He always lived in the countryside; built the houses that his family lived in; and still has a vegetable garden, cuts his own wood, carries it, and stacks it in a shed to be used for heating the house. Not only is the man on the move all the time, but he is also a voracious reader and active writer. Upon his return from the war, he got in the habit of writing a daily note, and I recently had the privilege of reading some of these journals, which spanned decades. He always starts his note with an observation on the weather, then a note on any wildlife he may have seen on his outings, a comment about what is going on in society around him, locally and nationally, followed by a personal note about what is going on with him and his family. The readings are fascinating because they cover so many years of personal, local, and national history. He still displays an impressively sharp mind. He is ready to engage me in discussion on any topic in the news or the family. The messages his life provides are captured in this book: Read. Write. Keep your brain active. Remain physically on the move.

The parents of a colleague live far from my father-in-law, on the island of Corsica, where the terrain rises sharply from the sea. My colleague's aging mother has to climb several flights of stairs to get to her house and descend them if she needs to do any shopping. Recently it was suggested that she move households to a lower dwelling so she wouldn't have to climb up and down so many stairs. She responded with wonderful insight and said, "Going up and down all these stairs is what is keeping my body alive and my mind sharp."

Not only are there these notable individuals who have combined longevity of life with intellectual lucidity, but many studies of societies or groups of individuals have made correlations between mental abilities and lifelong activities and habits. My own observations, combined with the messages that have come to us from these studies, lead to a very clear message that was eloquently articulated by Dr. Robert Wilson, who led the Baltimore Longitudinal Study of Aging. He put it this way: "The brain that we have in old age depends in part on what we ask it to do throughout life."[2]

That thinking changes things drastically. It used to be that when an older neighbour or friend had dementia, we thought they had Alzheimer's disease, meaning there was not much they could have done to avoid that outcome. It was their fate. Now we know that Alzheimer's disease is but one cause of dementia, and not the major one. In fact, we control a major part of how we age. And that is a good thing, because there is no consistent evidence of benefit from any pharmacologic agent in preventing or slowing cognitive decline due to Alzheimer's disease. The best thing is to avoid the awful condition of dementia before it starts, or slow it down before it progresses too far—and you have the power to do that.

Your Brain Is Modifiable

In addition to individual stories like my father-in-law's and my colleague's mother, the conclusion that we can reduce our chances of having dementia is supported by several large and informative studies. The Scottish Lothian study tested 70,000 children at age 11 and followed them over the years. The Lothian study showed clear evidence, perhaps not surprisingly, that the more intelligent a child was at age 11 the more likely it was for his or her cognitive abilities such as memory to be preserved in old age.[3] Genetics—who you picked for Mom and Dad—does play an important role, but that study also clearly showed that the participants' scores on IQ tests at the age of 11 predicted their score in old age less than 50% of the time. Most of how well a participant functioned in old age depended on what he or she did with the brain qualities they were provided at birth. So your mental function in old age is not written in stone—it is written in brainpower you can boost or waste, confirming the important concept of brain plasticity, meaning that your brain is malleable and modifiable. In confirmation of that statement, the study suggests that regardless of how smart the young Scots were at birth, those who remained physically fit, maintained their bilingual backgrounds by nurturing their knowledge of both Gaelic and English, acquired more education, and did not smoke had better test scores in old age than would have been expected. In other words, the years will take a different toll on the brain depending on what you did with what you were given.

Closer to home in Baltimore, the Longitudinal Study of Aging has enrolled almost 1,000 people over the past 50 years. Every two years they are retested using a battery of cognitive and physical tests and answer questionnaires on their past and current intellectual lifestyle, including whether they read books or write letters. Their brains are also examined after death. The researchers recently concluded that the thinking, memory, and other cognitive abilities of those who kept their brains busy as they aged were more preserved than those who had not.[4]

Combined, the observations from these studies are answering the question of why some individuals seem not only to live long but also maintain their cognitive functions at a very sharp level throughout life, whereas others seem to complain of "brain fog" at a young age. What do you have to do to belong firmly in the first category? This book will be answering these questions for you.

How Do We Think and Remember?

The richness of the information each of the 100 billion neurons in our brain receives and sends out is to some extent predetermined—it's inherited through genetics, which determine the number and quality of the neurons, other brain cells, and their connections, as well as the chemical environment they live in. So some of our cognitive and thinking abilities are not under our control, but the more important cues provided to the neurons in our brains are those acquired through our own activities and emotional environment. The trillions of contact points among the cells in the brain are known as synapses. At five months of gestation, the fetus has all the cells in the brain that he or she will have as an adult. The growth in the volume of the brain from then on is entirely due to the growth of the connections the neurons make on the receiving and outgoing ends. Keeping all these connections active and healthy is what provides us with the ability to think rapidly, calculate, recognize a familiar face, and remember an event, a date, or a place.

It is important to keep in mind something that has been known for a long time: that everything we do, or don't do, affects the health of these cells and their connections.[5] Their numbers and functions change with time but, more importantly, respond to the health of our bodies and to all our activities, be they physical, social, intellectual, emotional, or dietary.

Cells communicate through electrical impulses, which require chemical reactions to occur within and around the cells, and all this activity needs a lot of energy supplied rapidly. This is what makes the brain so dependent on its blood supply. It is estimated that the adult brain contains 600 km of blood vessels. That is more blood supply per unit weight than any other body organ. The brain does not store energy so it needs to receive a constant supply of it. Whether you are awake or sleeping, daydreaming or calculating, lying down or jogging, a variable but appropriate amount of energy is passed to the brain from the blood. If the blood supply to any brain region falls below the needed level, a blackout will occur, and in time this will translate into difficulties with thinking, memory, and other cognitive functions. This book will explain how to preserve the brain's blood supply to protect this hungry organ's access to needed energy.

In order for us to rapidly access information, evolution has assigned jobs to different brain parts. It is estimated that each brain region that is assigned a specific job receives and integrates information from 55 other brain regions before it sends out an action signal down the axon. Cognition, thinking, and memory are such important functions that many parts of the brain are involved in serving these functions. Still, in the same way that specific parts of the brain are dedicated to moving our arm or leg, providing us with the ability to see, and helping us keep our balance, certain parts of the brain carry the major burden of helping us remember, develop good judgement, and behave in appropriate ways. These complex activities require and access a number of structures we will review, but in order to make sense of the roles these structures play, let us review the different kinds of memories and other cognitive functions our brains perform.

How Many Kinds of Memories Are Stored in Our Brain?

It is truly amazing to think of the vast array of facts we carry in our heads. You not only remember facts about yourself (date of birth, age, names and histories of family members) and about the world around you (you know that Paris is the capital of France...), but you also remember how to get from home to work, where your favourite coffee shop is, how to get to it, and how to ride a bicycle. Scientists have given names to these different memory pools. Declarative or explicit memories refer to your ability to state a fact from memory: either an episodic memory (I hosted four people for supper last Thursday) or a semantic memory (John A. Macdonald was Canada's first prime minister). Non-declarative memories—things we remember how to do automatically and without conscious thought—refer to skills or abilities we remember and can undertake any time, such as reading, writing, singing. Yes, it takes memory to speak correctly and sing in tune. The reason scientists have made these distinctions is that the brain deals differently with information we are sending it, depending on whether we are learning a skill or learning a fact, and how important it is.

One very important part of our memory-storage system is embedded deep in our brain and is called the limbic system. It includes a number of structures that are vital for our memory functions. Parts of this limbic system are super-specialized. Recording and registering information have been assigned to a limbic system region of the brain called the hippocampus. This is the brain region that receives an explicit fact as soon as it is formed and, depending on how important it is for you to retain the fact and for how long, may convert the information from short-term to long-term memory. If the memory is needed for only a short while, the hippocampus will store it for you. As time passes, the hippocampus has to decide, based on input from you, if this memory is worth storing. If it is important, the hippocampus ships the memory out to other brain regions responsible for storing information, so that it can dedicate itself to storing additional new or recent memory. We know this because interrupting the activity of the hippocampus impairs recent but not remote memory.[6]

The yardstick the hippocampus uses to decide whether to store a memory long-term or not has to do with the emotional importance of the facts involved. Thus, it is possible to observe a person with impaired recent memory due to hippocampal damage break out into song when presented with music they heard in their youth. That is because despite the hippocampus being impaired, the memories that were already stored in areas like the temporal lobe can still be recalled. We have confirmed this relationship between old and recent memories because diseases or injuries that weaken or destroy the hippocampus may make storage of new memories difficult or impossible but still allow older memories to be recalled. Other observations have shown that even if the hippocampus remains intact, damage to structures it is connected to, such as the thalamus or temporal lobes, may result in memory deficits. It works in the other direction too: long-forgotten memories can be recalled if the temporal lobes are selectively activated.

Memory Function and Damage to the Hippocampus or Its Connections

When I did my neurology residency and later was on staff at the Montreal Neurological Institute, I had many opportunities to interact with Dr. Brenda Milner and listen to her lectures. Dr. Milner is still an active and productive neuropsychologist at the age of 96, and she recently received the Kavli Prize for the discovery of specialized brain networks for memory and cognition. She wrote a great deal on one patient, referred to as H.M., who underwent extensive brain surgery to cure his intractable epilepsy. The surgery included removal of major parts of the hippocampus on both sides. While H.M. was able to learn new tasks that Dr. Milner taught him (he had some procedural memory preserved), he could not remember interacting with her at all—it was as if every visit by her was the first one.[7]

Nature also provided an unfortunate experiment that confirmed more recently what we learned from H.M. about the role of the hippocampus in memory function. In late 1987, 150 individuals were poisoned when they consumed mussels contaminated with a naturally occurring toxin called domoic acid.[8] Four of these individuals died. One-third of the people who consumed these toxic mussels suffered neurologic abnormalities, and 14 of the most severely affected individuals were examined extensively. All had become confused and disoriented within 48 hours of eating the mussels, and it took some of them up to 12 weeks to recover, only to realize they had developed serious memory problems. Their other cognitive functions such as IQ, language ability, and emotional control were mostly intact, but they all suffered from amnesia. If you gave them a sentence and asked them to repeat it immediately, they were able to do so, but if you let some time go by and asked them again, it was impossible for them to come up with it. They had what we call anterograde amnesia, the same variety that H.M. suffered. The most severely affected individuals also had retrograde amnesia: they could not dredge up from memory important past events in their lives.

Where was the trouble? It was in the hippocampus and its neighbour, the amygdala, on both the right and left sides of the brain. Although these structures appeared normal on MRI scans, they were not consuming anywhere near normal amounts of energy when studied by other methods such as positron emission tomography, or PET, implying that brain cells within these structures had been poisoned to death.[9] This unfortunate experiment by nature confirmed the important role a healthy hippocampus plays in serving our memory functions. It also raised the level of oversight on mussels, so they remain one of my special culinary pleasures.

Colleagues in Japan have recently reported memory impairment in a 56-year-old man who suffered a ruptured brain aneurysm that destroyed his left hippocampus.[10] The patient showed no problems with movement, language, or sensation, but he had no memory of the sudden event that had brought him to hospital or of the events that had occurred since his hospitalization. As soon as a conversation with anyone ended, it was gone, even though it had been a normal conversation. The patient had no difficulty dredging up old memories, but could not form new ones.

So the hippocampus is a vital structure for our memory functions.

Cognitive Functions Beyond the Hippocampus

Despite the emphasis put here on the role of the limbic system and the hippocampus, we need to appreciate that multiple brain structures and regions play a role in our memory function and influence our judgement, behaviour, and other cognitive functions. Evidence for this comes from a variety of additional observations. Stimulation of parts of the amygdala, during surgery for instance, produces rage reactions that arise from fear, or the individual will mimic eating behaviour. As well in this setting, hormones will be produced, and blood pressure (BP) will rise. This shows us how our memory systems are connected with so many other functions, including emotions, everyday activities, and both wilful and automatic behaviour. Further evidence for the importance of memory function has come from accidents or surgeries that affected the temporal lobes or other parts of the limbic system. Thus, when the temporal lobes are damaged, not only will there be severe memory deficits, but the affected individual may also show a number of behavioural abnormalities, including depression, episodic violence, and sexual dysfunction.

A part of the brain called the prefrontal cortex is often referred to by neuroscientists as the CEO of the brain because that is the region we use to make rapid decisions that determine how we behave. The frontal lobe allocates our attention to what is most relevant at that moment. If memory is affected, the decisions may become delayed, unreliable, or unconventional. So it is important to recognize that not only is the limbic system involved in memory functions, it is also integrated into brain systems that mediate behaviour and emotional output, and may even be connected to systems that control our physical functions, like blood pressure and heart rate.

Let me give you another example of how memory is interconnected with and influences our behaviour. You are walking down the street. Even though you are not consciously aware of it, your brain is constantly scanning your environment. We refer to this as "scene processing," something your brain is doing all the time. Suddenly, it pays attention and alerts you that you may recognize someone coming down the street. As she gets closer, you recognize her either as a friend or someone you don't like. Whoa! Think about that. First, your brain activated a process known as selective attention, captured an image of the individual in the part of the brain that serves vision, which is in the occipital lobe in the back of the brain, and sent the information to the hippocampus. If you had seen this person recently, her face may still be embedded in the hippocampus, or if it has been a while, the information may exist only in more remote cortical regions. Regardless, the message of recognition that comes out is sent to the emotional centres of the brain for confirmation. The prefrontal cortex, the CEO of the brain, takes all this information in and makes an executive decision: Am I going to smile at this individual because I recognize a friend, or am I going to try to avoid her? Should I turn tail and run away because I recognize an enemy? If the decision is to run away, the information goes to the centres in the brain that control blood pressure and heart rate and send energy to your legs so that you can run. Although we are not fully aware of these reactions in our brains, you can imagine how any disruption in this system, for whatever reason, will potentially result in tragic consequences.

A patient came to see me recently very upset at the fact that his mother, who was suffering from dementia and resided in an old age home, looked at him when he went to visit her and asked him who he was! One can imagine that her visual functions were intact—she did see him—but when the visual information was sent to the hippocampus or beyond, the previously stored image of the son had disappeared due to her condition, resulting in no confirmation of familiarity. He felt devastated. You can see how, with dementia, the afflicted person is not the only one who suffers.

Information is transferred across the brain very rapidly. In the example of running into a person and recognizing their familiarity, the whole business might take less than milliseconds to complete. You might think that sending information through the thousands of connections each cell has would be slow and tedious, and you would be right, except for the fact that the brain has developed a rapid transit system. The message gets there rapidly because it hops across myelinated axons rapidly. An axon is a long, thready part of a nerve cell that sends out an electrical signal, or message, prompting an action. The message goes to its target cells, but because it has to get there rapidly, the axons are covered with a fatty substance called myelin that is ideally organized for rapid transmission. Instead of the message having to crawl through the axon itself, myelin allows the electrical message to jump across major segments of the axon to get to the target at lightning speed. Additionally, the brain has evolved so that the neurons are mostly lined up in the undulating outer layer of the brain, called cortex or grey matter, and all the myelinated axons are in the deeper white matter, which gets its name from the fact that myelin is lighter in colour. Figure 1 is an MRI scan showing the layering of the grey matter in a ribbon in the outer layers and the white matter more centrally.

If you think of the neurons as telephones, the myelinated axons are the telephone lines. Transmission through the axons occurs extremely rapidly so long as these myelinated axons remain healthy, and they serve not only our memory function but also other elements that combine to form what we generally refer to as personality: intact judgement, appropriate emotional control, an appreciation of self, imagination, foresight, and many more characteristics and functions. So, while memory is at the centre of our cognitive functions, collectively these functions harness the energies of major parts of our brain. When memory is impaired, our personalities also change.

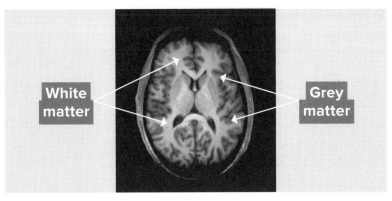

FIGURE 1

MRI of a normal brain, showing white and grey matter structures

So get ready! You now know enough about the brain to start tackling, and hopefully following, the rules that will allow you to protect your brain against dementia.

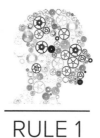

RULE 1

Grow Your Brain's Capacity for Cognitive Functions

Have you saved for a rainy day? You probably have because you thought some day you would need money to deal with an emergency. We all would like to feel financially secure in our old age too, so I suspect you would agree that a reserve fund for our retirement would be very useful. We would call on it when we needed to spend for a function or a project.

It is essentially the same simple principle that governs our brain's cognitive ability. You build a reserve of ability to think and remember so you can face future negative influences on your mind. In this regard, a very important study that has taught us a lot has been the Nun Study.[1] Essentially, 678 nuns of Notre Dame Congregation in the United States allowed scientists to test their ability to think, to evaluate their judgement, and to measure their memory functions. They also allowed the scientists to look into their early educational and family backgrounds, their early writing styles, and the richness of their written compositions; they even permitted the examination of their brains after death. The findings were startling: in many cases of individuals with totally normal memory and other cognitive functions during life and excellent test scores, their brains upon death showed great similarities to the pathology attributed to Alzheimer's disease. This implied that some individuals could think and remember and function cognitively very well as they aged despite a great deal of Alzheimer's disease found in their brains at autopsy. Importantly, the study was also able to correlate writing styles and richness of content in the early compositions, particularly the richness of phraseology and imagination in writing, with subsequent protection from dementia onset. In other words, genetic predisposition, who your mom and dad were, is an important determinant of how well you will age, but even more important is building, growing, and replenishing your cognitive reserve from an early age. The Nun Study emphasized the vital importance of starting to build your cognitive reserve early in life and maintaining it as you age.

With this information, scientists went to work to answer the questions "Why is it that there is this disconnect between the ability of some individuals to continue functioning normally in life, with normal mental and cognitive functions, even when their brains are invaded by Alzheimer's disease? How can you continue to think normally in the face of a deteriorating brain that has the hallmarks of this disease we all associate with dementia?" This was the genesis of the concept of cognitive reserve that constitutes Rule 1: you save when you are young—you build mental capacity in your early years and continue to replenish it throughout your life, so you can face the damaging conditions that are bound to come your way as you get older, including the accumulation of the nasty proteins of Alzheimer's disease, and overcome their negative impact on your thinking and memory functions. Clearly, despite the ravages of disease obvious on brain examinations, some individuals had overcome this barrier to normal mental function by building up, constantly replenishing, and incorporating intellectual reserve capacity into the structures of their brains as early as possible. These individuals were able to successfully call on these reserves to override the damage caused by disease and, despite it, function normally. When memory started to weaken, the severity of the decline was vastly different between two individuals whose brains showed similar degrees of abnormalities, again due to the variation in what they had done with what remained of their cognitive reserve capacities.

Before we go further, let us define cognitive ability. The word "cognitive" refers to all the activities our mind performs and the characteristics of our thinking abilities. "Cognition" includes our ability to perform the following mental activities:

- ▸ Remember facts, people, and places

- ▸ Pay selective attention to an event or a task

- ▸ Concentrate on the activity we are involved in

- ▸ Form good judgements about a situation

- ▸ Make reasonable decisions and execute them

- ▸ Be oriented in time and place

- ▸ Be able to connect memories sequentially and accurately

- ▸ Remember what an object we saw looks like when we are not looking at it

▸ Use language fluently, both when we speak it and when we process what we hear

▸ Calculate accurately

This list does not do justice to the complexities of our mind, however. For instance, memory is further defined as short term—lasting a matter of minutes—and long term, which appears to be limitless in its duration. This afternoon you will still be able to remember details of your morning, but that may not be the case a week from now. To be able to do so requires long-term memory, which implies the ability to store important information in our brain for a long time and be able to access it effortlessly.

How much brainpower you have in reserve with which to counter brain wear and tear over the years and still function well is known as "cognitive reserve." Cognitive reserve is defined as your ability to do more with your brain than one would predict from objectively assessing—say, by looking at a scan of your brain—the wear and tear your brain has sustained over the years. And there are multiple actions and measures you must take to build up your cognitive reserve. You will become familiar with all of them as you read this book. There are also multiple ways by which these reserves can be spent or become diminished as this book describes, and how fast your reserves are drained will determine how rapidly you develop cognitive difficulties.

Protecting and Promoting Our Cognitive Functions

Our ability to think normally depends on the richness of the connections among the action cells in our brain, called neurons.

It is estimated that each of the 100 billion neurons in the brain connects with as many as 1,000 other neurons. The neurons conduct electrical and chemical impulses to communicate not just with each other but also with organs outside the brain, like our muscles and the glands in our body. In addition to connecting directly with 1,000 other neurons, each neuron also communicates with as many as 30,000 other cells in the brain, in a process that is extremely precise. Thus, our brain is made up of an extensive communication network responsible for all our actions, feelings, and thoughts.

Each neuron in our brain is ideally shaped to do its job of both receiving information and transmitting it. On the receiving end, the neuron has tentacles that gather information from other cells and from its immediate environment. On the other end, the axon, covered with myelin, rapidly transmits the information to its neighbours.

You can see that the brain has to stay busy keeping alive and healthy the billions of connections necessary for us to enjoy normal mental functions. Under normal circumstances, even though you may not be aware of it, you are the boss: you are determining which connections among the billions of neurons in your brain are going to be preserved, and which ones are going to be let go. If you read a lot, the connections along the pathway from your brain's vision centres to the language comprehension centres will strengthen and over time will be in top shape. If you have read a new novel or started to learn a few words in a new language, those parts of the brain you have activated will be protected and promoted, and new connections will be made in the areas your actions stimulated. If you write a lot, the connections that will be kept in good shape are those that go from speech production centres in the brain to the fine motor control centres that allow your hand to make precise writing or typing motions. The connections from your vision centres back to your language centres will check to make sure what you write makes sense. The connections you activate will get increased blood supply and the ones you do not activate, the ones you ignore, will be gradually turned down and eventually turned off. How does that work? It is simple: the activity in your nerve cells is what determines if new blood vessels will be formed to supply energy to the region you have activated. So you are the ultimate decision-maker in what brain region serving which activity will thrive and remain healthy, and what region or activity will weaken and wither away. The brain is not going to waste energy maintaining connections among neurons you are not using. The richness and vitality of the connections and functions you establish in your brain are what constitute your cognitive reserve. That is what allows you to continue functioning normally even in the face of factors or disease conditions that could impair function. So it is important to restate Dr. Robert Wilson's saying: the brain we have in old age is the one we sculpted in our early and middle years by keeping the environment where the neurons exist healthy and by activating the brain circuits that will serve us in old age.

Nor does the mind reside separately and independently from what happens in our brain and the health conditions that prevail in the rest of our body. The brain is the master organ, and it is there to serve us, but to do that well it continuously senses and monitors everything inside you and around you: your cholesterol level, your sugar level, your salt intake, whether you have been physically active, had a good night's sleep or woke up several times, and what your mood has been lately—whether you are happy, sad, or depressed. In response to all these inputs, the brain activates cells, hormones, and chemicals; promotes the formation of new connections and preserves them; or suppresses others, all with significant consequences to your overall mental health.

Can I Continue to Grow My Cognitive Reserve?

The answer would appear to be a resounding yes. We've seen that cognitive reserve is based on the richness of the connections among brain cells, and while time makes it more difficult to create new brain connections and preserve them, there is plenty of evidence that it is possible, at any age, to create new brain connections and increase their resistance to the ravages of time. However, it is best to build cognitive reserve capacity early in life and keep at it as you get older. The medical literature suggests that what we do in our early and middle years with our brains—good or bad—has a major impact on our cognitive abilities in later life. Consequently, the earlier you follow the advice in this book, the better chance you stand of preserving brain and mind functions. *But it is never too late.* You and your brain never cross a point of no return for enhancing and growing your intellectual and cognitive functions.

Three important points are made by experts in cognitive reserve:

The first is that the brain likes variety. Exercising one part of your brain again and again does not necessarily result in activation of other parts and improvement of their functions. The brain is extremely efficient in the functions it activates in response to mental exercises, for instance, so we must vary the input. Think of it this way: if someone is a good hockey player, it doesn't necessarily make them a good tennis player. However, the strong muscles developed playing hockey will be useful while practising tennis. Doing one thing repeatedly for a long time is not as useful to your brain or effective for your mental functions as doing many things for shorter periods of time. So do not spend all your time doing one thing again and again.

The second important point is that the brain likes and needs to be pushed. What you demand of it must overcome its natural desire to preserve energy and take it easy! Plasticity of the brain, meaning its ability to develop new skills and improve thinking and memory functions, serves you best when you push it. As an older adult, you have all of life's experiences to work for you, and they have promoted your brain's plasticity. So while you can take full advantage of that, you cannot stop making new demands on the brain.

The third important point is that some "forgetting" is normal. In addition to fixed memories, there are items you remembered for a while but "voluntarily" forgot: for a long time you could remember the details of that horrible car accident you saw happening in front of you 12 years ago, but the details are now blurred. And this is an important point to stress: forgetting information that is not "important," that doesn't have survival value or emotional impact for you, is a normal process. Your brain prioritizes not only what needs to be stored as memory but also what can be safely discarded because it is not essential. After a hectic morning, don't be upset if you do not remember at the end of the day where your car is in the parking lot.

Will Brain Games Build My Cognitive Reserve?

I get asked this question quite frequently, and my answer is nuanced. A lot of people appear convinced that brain games will ward off the threat of dementia. Unfortunately, the evidence for this is not very strong, nowhere near as strong as it is for the benefit to our minds of physical activity. A recent article in *Neurology* described a study involving more than 600 men and women, average age 70, that compared the relative impact of physical exercise and mental activities on the brain's structure. The participants' MRI brain scans were examined over a three-year period. The research showed that social and intellectual activities did not appear to provide as much benefit to the structural health of the participants' brains as did regular physical exercise. The group that kept moving and stayed physically active experienced less brain shrinkage and less damage to the brain's wiring than the group that sat a lot but did a lot of "thinking" exercises.[2] Interestingly, if the activity was complex and demanded multiple tasks, such as playing a video game for 30 minutes daily, the participants grew more grey matter in the brain areas associated with spatial navigation, strategic planning, working memory, and motor performance. However, the next year the same journal published the results of a study involving a different group of 294 people. As in the Nun Study, these individuals were given an annual test measuring memory and thinking and their brains were studied after death. The conclusion of this study was that those who had a record of keeping their brains busy had slowed their cognitive decline compared to those who let their brains idle.[3] So it appears that the more varied and demanding the activities you challenge your brain with are, the better your intellectual and cognitive abilities will be. A crucial requirement for maintaining cognitive abilities in top shape seems to be physical activity and avoiding a sedentary lifestyle.

Many people have taken up brain exercises. Economists have estimated that the total revenues from sales of programs and tools to "exercise" the brain exceeded $1 billion for the first time in 2012, thanks in large part to the rapid growth of consumer firms such as Lumosity, a brain-training company that provides online games for improvng your memory and problem solving. There is still debate as to whether these brain exercises are effective in preserving memory function and building cognitive reserve. A recent study found that 12 weeks of Lumosity training improved executive brain functions in a group of women.[4] Another study of the impact of Lumosity on brain function was tested by both formal cognitive testing and functional MRI. Fifty Canadians performed brain exercises suggested by Lumosity for one month, with tests being performed both before and after this period of brain training, and the conclusion was that one month of Lumosity made little difference to either cognitive testing or the connectivity and efficiency of brain function judged by functional MRI studies (fMRI).[5] This confirmed previous evidence that brain training does not transfer to untrained tasks.

So the yin-yang of cognitive reserve is this: on the one hand, you use it or you lose it, and on the other hand the brain is very parsimonious and will not expend energy making new connections and maintaining them every time you put it to work. The brain wants to know that you are serious, meaning that it will go to work and set up new connections or confirm and enrich ones that are already there only if the mental activity you are imposing is persistent and emotionally meaningful.

Many examples from real life confirm this finding. Cabbies in London, England, are taught, over a four-year period, the names of streets in their city and are rigorously tested for their navigational knowledge. MRI examinations of their brains show that the brain parts that deal with navigation and orientation in space, including the hippocampus, are larger in the cabbies than in the rest of us. Other parts of their brains remain normal in size. Similarly, the brains of musicians and artists are modified in the areas that serve their skills. The corollary for you is that putting your mind to work, say with repeated Sudoku games, will not hurt your brain. Indeed, the part of the brain that provides you with the skills you need to do Sudoku may even grow in size, but it will not necessarily improve your overall memory functions. You will be a good Sudoku player, and that's it. The brain will not expend energy to improve your judgement or your sense of humour just because you worked it hard playing Sudoku. Stephen Kosslyn, until recently the director of Stanford's Centre for Advanced Study in the Behavioural Sciences, agrees with the brain's parsimony. He says: "The shocking truth is that the opportunities to generalise are very limited. If you practise some cognitive task you are basically practising that thing. If something else is very similar in its underlying structure there may be some transferability, but rarely 100%."

Here are some suggestions to grow your brain's cognitive reserve and protect your thinking and memory:

1. Playing brain games is not a waste of time, but the benefit is limited.

2. Keep varying how you activate your brain. Demand multiple kinds of brain activities, especially ones that require eye–hand coordination such as playing tennis or playing some video games, or eye–ear–body coordination such as dancing to music.

3. Continue to read and to write, do calculations, complete crossword puzzles, put together multi-piece picture puzzles, commit telephone numbers and other information to memory—in short, keep that brain working by performing many tasks, and do so repeatedly.

4. Do not allow your brain to tune out by watching a lot of TV. Watching TV is usually a passive activity that does not stimulate the brain.

5. Remain socially engaged. Make sure you have good friends who care about you, and vice versa, and connect with them frequently.

6. Keep physically active. Go for walks if you can, and if you enjoy swimming, it is a great way to stay cool while working out.

7. Do not get discouraged and give up if you have an occasional memory lapse. Keep at it.

Later in the book, I describe the activities you need to do, and those you need to avoid, to stay sharp. And here is the crux of the story that relates memory to lifestyle and other activities. Because memory is so crucial for human activity, new neurons are continuously generated and deposited in the hippocampus, the brain structure that is crucial for memory function. Other brain regions do get the same upkeep but, as far as we know, not to the same extent. That makes the hippocampus, a central structure for our memory functions, a very privileged part of the brain. Nature has set up this whole system to renew the cells that are used up in the hippocampus by depositing new stem cells that get integrated into the circuitry of this structure. It is important to remember, however, that the recruitment of new neurons to the brain, called neurogenesis, is only the first step. These neurons now have to integrate into brain circuits in order to rejuvenate pre-existing lines of communication (neuronal pathways), and that requires energy expenditure and a healthy brain environment. Even in old age when our cognitive faculties tend to diminish, the hippocampus constantly renews and rebuilds itself. But the brain does nothing it does not have to do, hence the need to constantly encourage new cell formation and integration into our memory circuits. Our "plastic" brain can be sculpted, and the sculptor is you.[6]

Symptoms of Cognitive Decline: The Case of Mrs. V.B.

What happens when our cognitive reserve diminishes or gets used up? We develop symptoms. Initially, the symptoms are limited to memory lapses that are not serious—they are not sufficient to interfere with the ability to function at work or at home. This stage is referred to as mild cognitive impairment (MCI). The diagnosis of full-blown dementia is made when thinking, memory, or decision-making (executive) difficulties begin to interfere with the activities and enjoyment of life.

Three years ago, Mrs. V.B. came to my office with her adult daughter. She was 68 years old then and lived in a condo by herself. Her husband had died four years earlier. She and her husband used to enjoy going dancing, which they usually did with their friends, but following the death of her husband, many friends had failed to include Mrs. B. in their activities, and she gradually lost her social contacts. She had three children, two of whom lived not far from her and checked on her regularly.

For about a year prior to their visit with me, the daughters had noticed their mother's memory was declining. She would often invite her children and grandchildren for supper, but they began to notice that her cooking was slowly deteriorating. She would laugh it off, saying she was letting her imagination flourish. The visits were a real joy as Mrs. B. clearly loved her grandchildren and made special treats for them. She also talked about how she and other ladies in the condo where she lived went to a nearby coffee shop. On one occasion, one of Mrs. B.'s daughters had gone to the coffee shop with her and indeed Mrs. B. was welcomed by her first name. Thus, despite some issues, Mrs. B. was functioning well. The daughters had chatted with the neighbours and left them their phone numbers in case of emergency or need.

When I had examined Mrs. B., the results were normal. She was 5'10" and weighed 138 pounds. Her waist circumference was 85 cm and her blood pressure at rest was 140/90 mmHg (blood pressure is measured in millimetres of mercury, which has the symbol Hg; at rest blood pressure should not exceed 120/80). The neurological exam was normal. I had conducted a Montreal Cognitive Assessment (MoCA) test with her and she had scored 24 out of 30, right where I would expect someone with mild cognitive impairment to be. The MoCA test is a screening tool of cognition used by clinicians to provide a brief overview of cognitive abilities.

Because the medical literature shows that MCI can occasionally be a reversible consequence of infections, thyroid malfunction, alcoholism or alcohol withdrawal, vitamin deficiencies, or a small stroke, I checked out all these possibilities and eliminated them. Because Mrs. B. had said "I love my salt" and her blood pressure was 10 to 20 mmHg too high for my comfort, I advised Mrs. B. to cut down on her salt intake.

Now Mrs. B.'s family physician was asking me to see the patient again. The current visit was precipitated by the fact that at their last encounter with Mrs. B., her children had noted that she had used very unusual ingredients in a salad she prepared, adding tomato sauce to the salad instead of dressing. They also noticed that her kitchen, which was previously impeccably clean, had deteriorated. When she set the table, the dishes had stains and smudges. As well, they noted that her personal hygiene had deteriorated. She had a faint smell of someone who did not bathe regularly. On a separate visit she could not remember the name of one of her grandchildren. The daughter told me Mrs. B. had become an avid TV watcher. Then one day a neighbour called the daughter to say Mrs. B. wanted to go for their regular coffee in her nightgown, and even though it was winter, she didn't think she needed a coat. On another occasion, the daughters received a call from the police because they had found Mrs. B. wandering the street looking for a coffee shop.

In my office, I saw that Mrs. B. had changed significantly. She was more unkempt and smelled slightly, and although she recognized me and greeted me, she wanted to know if I liked my new office even though I had not moved. Her examination showed she had lost 12 pounds in the three years since her last visit, and her blood pressure was now well above normal at 154/94 mmHg. Her neurological exam remained relatively intact but her MoCA test showed that her intellectual and cognitive capacity had deteriorated into dementia range. Her brain scan revealed small scars in the white matter of the brain, suggesting she had suffered small strokes.

I had a long discussion with Mrs. B. and her daughters. They understood the fact that Mom had deteriorated, was not managing her diet properly, and was increasingly isolated socially. They initially thought they could turn things around or at least stabilize the situation by visiting her daily. This was very hard on them, but despite the frequent visits, it rapidly became clear to them that Mrs. B. could not live alone in her condo anymore. For one thing, Mrs. B. was not reliably taking the BP medication she had been prescribed. She had to be placed in a home where there was round-the-clock care and supervision.

With the example of Mrs. B. in mind, let's look at a spectrum of memory lapses connected with one task: trying to come up with someone's name. A totally normal but busy, harried, and hassled individual may forget the name of a remote acquaintance, someone who is not a close work colleague or a family member, when she suddenly runs into this person. That would be considered normal. Often the name will come to them later on, sometimes as soon as the acquaintance has just gotten out of sight. Someone with MCI, however, may not remember the name of a close work partner when they run into them, and someone with dementia may not remember the name of one of their children or grandchildren.

Situations that would merit a diagnosis of mild cognitive impairment, or MCI, include misplacing objects or going to the kitchen and for a while not being able to remember what you needed there. You know your way to work and have never gotten lost, but when someone asks you how you get to work, you have trouble naming the streets you travel on. Importantly in MCI, people around you are not expressing concern about your memory difficulties, your work productivity, or your general ability to function without increased effort, help, or support. Individuals with MCI often make lists. When they want to remember something later, they write it down immediately and review the list periodically. They may put stickers here and there to jog their memories. The important distinction between MCI and something worse is that individuals with MCI do not have impaired judgement and their executive functions are intact. Their personalities do not change substantially, their sense of orientation continues to serve them well, and their ability to make appropriate decisions remains intact. Nonetheless, MCI is a warning sign that you need to connect with your physician to assess the problem, evaluate what medical risk factors may be affecting your brain function, and receive advice on what can be done to reverse the process.

When MCI morphs into dementia, the symptoms have considerably more impact on the individual's life and on the people around them. To be diagnosed with dementia, you must display a deficit in memory plus trouble in at least one other cognitive domain such as the ability to produce or interpret language, or make decisions in a timely fashion. As well, these deficits must reach the point of affecting daily functioning, meaning that the individual experiences difficulty performing familiar tasks. He or she has difficulty coming up with details of past events or information, even when they are reminded of them. Thus, they may gradually forget how to make toast or cook an egg, or they may ask for details on how to make a dish they used to be very familiar with. Even when reminded, there is no guarantee the right ingredients will be used or the dish will be a success. Individuals affected by dementia frequently become lost and disoriented. They may not remember where they live if taken out of their homes and could not give you directions on how to get there. Dementia almost always involves some difficulty in communication, either in understanding language or, more frequently, in producing it easily or intelligently. Dementia also diminishes good judgement and interferes with activities we refer to as executive functions: the ability to accomplish complex tasks that require some abstract thinking, like keeping a bank account accurately or preparing a multi-step meal.

As we have learned, dementia also frequently leads to a change in personality as the condition sweeps over parts of the brain that make us kind or help us suppress our anger at certain situations. The individual may have visual hallucinations whereby they tell you that someone you know is dead has come to visit them and they had a nice chat. The change in the personalities of the individuals affected may also involve increased suspiciousness of the people around them to the point of becoming paranoid. They may claim, for instance, that family members are stealing from them or intend to cause them harm.

Dementia usually also includes some disorientation. The affected person may not remember how to go from the kitchen to the bathroom even though they are in their own home. They may attempt to leave the house at night to look for someone, and as soon as they are out the door not remember where they live. They may also become uncoordinated so they may weave their way around the house, which increases their chances of falling and injuring themselves. Dementia can be destructive of so many aspects of the affected individual's mind that we can hardly recognize the person anymore.

Finally, individuals affected by dementia can also exhibit unusual behaviour. The type of behavioural, emotional, or cognitive symptoms will vary in those affected by this condition. Some may show more memory problems while others may exhibit more behavioural problems. They may lose their inhibitions. A colleague of mine whose mother had dementia had brought her to live with him. One evening when he was hosting several colleagues for supper, his mother came out of her room in her underwear and greeted everyone. He shepherded her back to her room and got her dressed. Demented individuals can also be very frustrated and angry, and may act on their feelings without inhibitions. Thus the affected individual may suddenly haul off and slap a person who is very dear to them over a trivial issue and feel no remorse or offer any apology.

Our Personality Resides in Our Brain Structures

Perhaps the most famous illustration of how our personality resides in our brain and is affected by memory is the case of Phineas Gage. He is often referred to as "the most famous patient in neurology."[7] In 1848 the 25-year-old Gage was a railroad foreman. He was using an iron rod to tamp down explosive powder when the powder detonated, and the rod went through his left cheek and straight up, tearing into his brain and flying out of his skull. His motor functions were sufficiently intact that he could walk to a nearby railroad cart and ask to be taken to a doctor. He had a rocky recovery, but thanks to Dr. John M. Harlow, he survived with intact motor functions and ability to walk and talk, but suffered severe changes to his personality. The part of his brain that had been damaged was the left prefrontal region, the area referred to as the CEO of the brain because of its role in helping us select some actions and inhibit others. The white matter in that region of Gage's brain was the most affected.

In 1868, Dr. Harlow described Gage's personality changes as follows: "He is fitful, irreverent, indulging at times in the grossest profanity (which was not previously his custom), manifesting but little deference for his fellows, impatient of restraint or advice when it conflicts with his desires, at times pertinaciously obstinate, yet capricious and vacillating, devising many plans of future operations, which are no sooner arranged than they are abandoned in turn for others appearing more feasible. A child in his intellectual capacity and manifestations, he has the animal passions of a strong man. Previous to his injury, although untrained in the schools, he possessed a well-balanced mind, and was looked upon by those who knew him as a shrewd, smart businessman, very energetic and persistent in executing all his plans of operation. In this regard, his mind was radically changed so decidedly that his friends and acquaintances said he was 'no longer Gage.'"

Reversible Causes of Memory Trouble

I referred to checking Mrs. B. for a number of reversible causes of dementia. Let's spend a moment talking about these.

Deficiency in a number of vitamins can cause memory difficulty, most prominently thiamine, or B1. This condition, frequently associated with poor nutrition, used to be seen in heavy drinkers and in other individuals who due to difficulties with digestion could not keep food down for some time. As thiamine levels fall, the brain becomes less able to use glucose, an essential source of energy. Sometimes a severely dehydrated patient is brought into the emergency room after being found passed out from excess alcohol consumption. An intravenous injection with fluid that contains glucose is started to rehydrate the patient and a syndrome called Wernicke-Korsakoff is precipitated. The patient becomes confused in addition to having double vision. He has anterograde memory deficit: if you walk into the room, introduce yourself, chat a little, then step out for a few minutes and come back in, it is like he's never met you. You are always somebody new. Often the memory deficit is associated with confabulations—incoherent stories the patient spins out, often combined with visual hallucinations. Many of these symptoms abate as soon as thiamine, 50 to 100 mg, is given intravenously or intramuscularly. Many an intern has called colleagues to come to the ER to see a case of Wernicke-Korsakoff, only to be embarrassed when they arrive to find a normal patient who has just received a B_1 shot.

Other vitamin deficiencies that must be ruled out as causes of memory difficulty are B_{12} and folate. These two vitamins are associated with the elevation in a protein called homocystein that has negative consequences on the health of our blood vessels.

Another reversible cause of dementia, hypothyroidism, is caused by a thyroid gland that is not putting out enough thyroid hormone. Patients whose thyroid gland is not producing enough of the hormone will initially suffer from mental slowing and apathy, but if the condition is not detected and corrected, full-blown dementia may be the outcome.

A condition known as normal pressure hydrocephalus can also cause memory and cognitive difficulty, usually associated with walking difficulty and incontinence. If the neurological history and exam raise this possibility, and the brain CT or MRI scan are compatible with this diagnosis, a test to check the flow dynamics of the cerebrospinal fluid (called a cisternogram) is needed. It is important to do all this because a relatively simple surgical procedure to introduce a shunt to drain the excess cerebrospinal fluid in a controlled fashion can often reverse the walking and memory problems.

Repetitive head trauma is now also recognized as a potential cause of eventual dementia and unfortunately, it is only preventable but not reversible. You are likely aware of the recent settlement between the National Football League and players who suffered repeated concussions and as a consequence have cognitive impairment. The brain is simply unforgiving of repeated jarring and sudden acceleration, deceleration, and rotation. There is a reason why of all the organs in the body, only your brain was put in a tight, strong, and rigid bony box.

You are not going to get dementia if you fall off your bike when you are not going too fast and are wearing a helmet, but if you are a boxer, you may suffer a condition known as pugilistic dementia, and if you are a football player who gets concussions or a soccer player who heads the ball too often and too vigorously, you may in time affect your brain's ability to think. This realization is now forcing us to reconsider how we play hockey, where fighting among players is still unfortunately valued as added entertainment, but the rules have to change because what we were cheering is potential injury to the players' mental health and cognitive abilities for the rest of their lives.

Finally, it is important to question individuals suffering from memory deficits about their prescribed or over-the-counter medications. The risk of dementia is higher in individuals who take high doses of drugs that block a neurotransmitter called acetylcholine over prolonged periods. These are usually drugs taken to treat allergies such as hay fever, pills that promote sleep, and drugs that treat urinary incontinence. Some drugs taken to treat depression can also have an anticholinergic impact.

Temporary Inability to Form Certain Memories

An example of this type of memory loss is the case of a man I'll call John, who was referred to me early in my career. He had been diagnosed in the ER with an episode of transient global amnesia (TGA). He was in his mid-40s, married with three children. He had always been a faithful husband and good father. But his marriage was undergoing some stresses and sex with his wife had become infrequent. When John's firm hired Jessie, an attractive single mother in her mid-30s, the two were brought together because of their jobs. One Saturday, John and Jessie met at the office to work on a project. After a successful completion of the task, they went out for dinner. When it was time to leave, Jessie was concerned about her ability to drive so John offered to follow behind her in his own car. During the drive, John had fantasies about having sex with Jessie—John's wife and children were away and Jessie's daughter was with her father, so the opportunity was there. He was aware his heart was pounding and he was sweating. When John got out of his car at the parking garage, he appeared disoriented, continually asking, "Where am I? What time is it?" After Jessie ascertained that John had not had a stroke, she suggested he go to the ER, saying she would drive behind him to ensure his safety. At the ER he was examined and diagnosed with a TGA.

This unusual situation teaches us a lot about the process of laying down new memories. During an episode of TGA, the patient is unable to lay down new memories, called anterograde amnesia, but they are completely conscious, fully communicative, and alert. They can drive and do other complex tasks. The problem seems to be that the specific part of the brain that lays down new memories is not functioning because it is not receiving enough blood supply to work well. This reduction in blood supply during TGA affects the hippocampus and the medial temporal region, and has been seen with severe anxiety, intensive physical activity, straining, acute pain, and, yes, intercourse. The symptoms last anywhere from one to eight hours before resolving. It has been suggested that the anxiety or the physical activity causes the release of a small blood clot from the heart or an artery, and its size is just right to block the vessel feeding the structures I listed, and eventually it goes through the region or breaks up, resulting in resolution of the symptoms.

How Are Cognitive Decline and Dementia Diagnosed?

The methods we use to diagnose mild cognitive impairment (MCI) and dementia are changing. The history that the patient or family members give to the doctor or the therapist regarding memory function, behaviour, and judgement is crucial for a conclusive diagnosis. There is an old saying in medicine that especially applies here: if you don't have a diagnosis by the end of the history you obtained from the patient and/or the caregiver, you will likely not have one after the exam—so the history one obtains in the clinic setting is crucial. Nonetheless, we have come a long way in having tools that allow us to make a firm diagnosis.

In the Nun Study, the individuals were administered several cognitive tests to assess their memory, judgement, executive functions, and personalities. Many of these tests are time-consuming and frequently overlap in their assessments of cognitive function. They also may not test specific spheres of cognition. Earlier, I referred to the Montreal Cognitive Assessment (MoCA) test—it has been a most welcome addition. It was developed in 1996 in Montreal by Dr. Ziad Nasreddine when he realized that taking 90 minutes to evaluate one patient's cognitive function was not compatible with an efficient neurological practice. Proving the saying that necessity is the mother of invention, he pioneered the tool we know as MoCA.[8] The test features 11 subtests that assess all mental processes—attention; concentration; executive functions, which include planning and organizing; memory; language—as well as skill at copying a figure given to you and coming up with the face of a clock that shows the time to be 10:50. MoCA also tests calculation, orientation, and conceptual thinking. The test should take less than 15 minutes to complete in the clinic or the office. (The MoCA test can be found online.) Its enormous advantage over other tests is not only that it is quick, but also that it identifies the cognitive spheres that may be in deficit, so that if possible something can be done about it.[9]

Prior to MoCA, the test most commonly used to assess cognitive function was the MMSE (the mini mental state examination). When MoCA and MMSE were compared, not only was MoCA much faster, but it was also better. It detected 90% of subjects with MCI when the MMSE picked only 18% of this group, and the MoCA detected 100% of subjects with dementia when MMSE could identify only 78% of them. For these reasons, MoCA was endorsed by an international conference held in 2005 jointly sponsored by the National Institutes of Health in the United States and the Canadian Stroke Network.

I want to emphasize that if an individual is seen to suffer from even mild cognitive or memory problems, he or she should consult with a physician. The reason is that mild problems with memory may progress to full-blown dementia, and the affected individual should be examined and tested for potentially reversible causes of memory difficulty and receive advice on how to counteract the problem. The clinician or health care provider will likely do a thorough general and neurological examination looking for possible contributing causes, order a brain CT scan or an MRI scan, and likely order some blood tests. These exams will allow the practitioner to assess general health, specific risk factors that may diminish cognitive health, and any impairment of neurologic function. Brain imaging allows us to visualize brain volume, assess if there is brain atrophy, and try to determine if strokes or other conditions that affect mental function are evident. More about that later.

Caregiving: One Person's Dementia Can Be a Vortex That Sucks in Many

I want to deal here with an aspect of dementia that is not often top of mind when a diagnosis is made. Dementia is a condition that frequently takes many years to progress to the stage of total dependency. If a loving, caring parent who has made sacrifices for the children, or a partner who has been a loving companion for years, begins to show memory difficulty, one or more family members may assume the responsibility of caregiving.

Caregiving is an act of love, but it is a very demanding one. The caregiver must have endless patience, an unlimited reserve of good humour, and a high level of stress tolerance. Even a caregiver hired for the job requires these qualities. The average lifespan of a person with dementia is seven years, but they can live for two decades in this state, so the caregiver can be in it for the long haul. It is estimated that 15 million people in the United States and more than 1 million Canadians are providing unpaid care for a parent, family member, or friend with dementia.

Caregivers face many challenges. They are often house-bound with the impaired individual. They have to be alert, day and night, to make sure that the individual will not do something bizarre and unexpected, like walk out of the house in the dead of night; sometimes the person just stepped out to get the newspaper from the mailbox or the porch and might not remember how to get back in, so the caregiver has to be constantly vigilant to such things. Dementia patients are often incontinent and may resist the attention needed to clean or bathe them. One of the biggest challenges faced by caregivers is dealing with an agitated person who can't be reasoned with, or one who is verbally or physically abusive. In addition, care providers frequently face isolation as the number of visitors dwindles.

For all these reasons, caregivers can become exhausted, depressed, or physically ill themselves. It is important to be sufficiently in touch with your feelings and state of health to face the difficult decision of placing in an institution someone who never abandoned you. Support groups can be crucially important as they provide an opportunity for sharing challenges with others and receiving friendship and advice. As well, in some jurisdictions, there are programs that provide respite, occasionally sufficient for the caregiver to be able to return to work.

An intact brain is necessary to preserve our memory but we need to push it so it doesn't become lazy. An intact brain is also essential to maintain our personality, help us make the right decisions in a timely fashion, and put a check on our antisocial impulses. An intact brain is essential if we want to remain who we are.

So far we have talked about the positive side of the cognitive reserve ledger. In the next chapters we are going to learn about the debit side of the cognitive reserve equation—all the things that can diminish your brain's reserve capacity and make you more vulnerable to dementia and how to avoid them or counter them. We will learn measures to take during our lifetime to build up the credit side of our cognitive reserve and diminish the drain on it. Get ready!

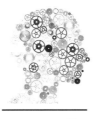

RULE 2

Reduce the Debit Calls on Your Mind

In the rest of this book, I will outline measures you can take to improve the credit–debit balance of your brain's cognitive abilities. What are the awful things that can happen to our brains that would diminish our cognitive reserve? These are what I put in the brain's debit column. How many of them are preventable, and how many of them are unavoidable? Keeping in mind that any interruption in brain circuitry, no matter how small, has the potential to impair one's ability to think, remember, or make appropriate judgements, let me outline some conditions that can lead to dementia and suggest whether they are preventable.

Brain Diseases We Can't Prevent That Can Lead to Dementia

Many patients who suffer from Parkinson's disease will have cognitive impairment and may eventually exhibit dementia.

Multiple sclerosis has a similar unfortunate impact on those who suffer from it. Aggressive cancers that invade the brain can also lead to dementia. These are three conditions we know a lot about but not enough to prevent them or diminish their unfortunate consequences on the patients' minds and cognitive functions.

A number of other less common conditions affect the brain and can lead to dementia. Frontotemporal degeneration, also called Pick's disease, results in the gradual atrophy (shrinkage) of the frontal and temporal lobes of the brain, areas that are essential for control of emotion, decision-making, and judgement. Although memory is not initially affected, the person suffering from frontotemporal dementia may become silent and apathetic and may develop odd behaviour, all consistent with dementia.

But the major unpreventable and so far untreatable condition that can lead to dementia is Alzheimer's disease. Alzheimer's disease is defined by two signature brain deposits that are seen when the brain is examined under the microscope in pathology. These are called plaques and tangles. Plaques look like stains on the brain. They are caused by deposits of a protein called β-amyloid in the blood vessels of the brain and in the brain itself. Tangles look like matted hair under the microscope, and when they are analyzed they turn out to be deposits of another protein called tau. Brain sections of the hippocampus region of the brain where these deposits abound, seen under low and high magnification revealing the plaques and tangles, are shown in Figure 2.

In a patient with severe Alzheimer's disease, an MRI scan is usually very instructive, as shown in Figure 3.

Think of these brain scans as showing a slice across the brain just above the ears. The convention is that brain images are

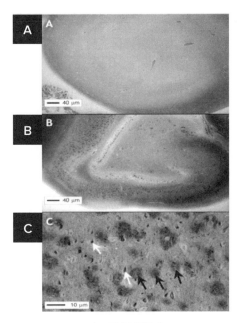

FIGURE 2

Images of a hippocampus

A. A normal hippocampus

B. A hippocampus of a patient with Alzheimer's disease (Bielschowsky stain) at low magnification. The numerous dark brown spots seen in the abnormal hippocampus are the plaques typical of Alzheimer's disease.

C. At higher magnification, these plaques are more visible (black arrows) and, in addition, tangles (white arrows) seen in Alzheimer's disease are also clearly visible.

projected as if you were looking at them from below, meaning that the part of the image that is on the viewer's left side is the right side of the scanned person's brain. The normal brain shown on the left of the figure fills the space inside the skull. The few black spots in the MRI of that normal brain are in

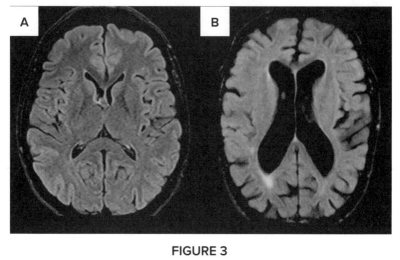

FIGURE 3

A. MRI scan of a normal brain

B. MRI scan of a patient with Alzheimer's disease: The brain is showing severe atrophy (shrinkage)

fact cerebrospinal fluid or CSF, which travels around in brain ventricles and bathes the brain. On the right is a scan of a person who has lost a lot of brain matter through the death of brain cells and their connections and has dementia. The space vacated by the brain that has shrunk is now filled with the expansion of the ventricles, hence those big black spaces filled with CSF in the middle of the figure. The thinning of the cortex and the enlarged ventricles in a patient suffering from dementia are hallmarks of Alzheimer's disease.

What Percentage of Dementia Is Caused by Alzheimer's Disease?

Most of the articles on this topic state that Alzheimer's disease is the major cause of dementia. There is also a tendency, even in the scientific literature, to refer to all dementias as Alzheimer's disease. The advent of brain imaging and improved correlations of dementia with other medical conditions have allowed us to re-examine this statement. There is now general agreement that another type of pathology or abnormality we call brain vascular disease can contribute to dementia in a major way. This is a disease of the blood vessels that feed the brain. The condition has very significant consequences for brain function, including the development of dementia. This new knowledge is allowing us to estimate the contribution of vascular disease to dementia in the population and is radically changing what we thought were the causes of dementia.

Two studies can help illustrate this. The first one, from 2006, showed how vascular risk factors have forced a reassessment of the causes of dementia, concluding that pure Alzheimer's disease is responsible for about 27% of dementias.[2] Thus the best estimate we have for dementia that is caused by a genetic predisposition to Alzheimer's disease alone is about a quarter of all dementias, the rest being due to pure vascular disease or a mixture of vascular disease and Alzheimer's disease. These figures for various causes of dementia were confirmed more recently.[3] The researchers used data in the National Alzheimer's Coordinating Center and compared the clinical information available on patients with what autopsy and neuropathology examination revealed. In patients with dementia who had been diagnosed with Alzheimer's disease, 79.9% showed abnormalities of the blood vessels in their brains and outside of it. They suffered from vascular disease. These findings show that a disease of blood vessels feeding the brain contributes to 75 to 80% of the dementias. The crucial implication of these studies is that prevention of vascular disease, particularly in early and middle life, represents the best chance we have to decrease our risk of dementia and delaying its onset. So let's look at what constitutes vascular disease and how we can prevent vascular disease of the brain.

Brain Vascular Diseases

Blood supply to the brain can be impaired at various levels and for varying reasons. When large arteries that feed the brain, such as the carotid arteries in your neck, develop thick walls that harden them, we call that atherosclerosis. The thicker walls make the blood vessels less flexible, and if the artery walls keep getting thicker and thicker, blood flowing to brain regions served by that artery can decline. When your doctor puts a stethoscope over your neck, he or she is listening for an unusual whooshing sound that can be heard if the blood is going through a constriction in your carotid artery. If the flow of blood falls below the brain's tolerance levels for more than four or five hours, the brain will sustain damage. When the hungry cells in the brain do not get the energy they need, the affected person suffers a stroke.

While narrowing of a large artery can be compensated for to some extent by dilation of other arteries overlapping the territory it supplies, narrowing of the smaller branch arteries, called arterioles, or damage to any of the even smaller penetrating blood vessels called capillaries may not be compensated for because they do not have buddy arteries (called collaterals) that can open up to make up for their closure. Thus occlusion of an arteriole or a penetrating blood vessel will result in a small area of damage to the brain, usually in the white matter, where the transmission lines from the neurons are bunched together.

If trouble in the structure of the brain is sufficiently extensive, it will have negative consequences on the ability of the individual to think clearly, to remember, and to make appropriate judgements. This is why the most prevalent form of cognitive impairment is due to vascular disease. Depending on its location and its severity, the vascular event may or may not be felt by the patient when it occurs, but it will almost certainly result in abnormalities on the examination, the imaging studies, or the cognitive evaluation that a physician will conduct.

The brain is unforgiving of vascular events.

Strokes: The Ones You Are Aware Of

Mrs. E.J. was a 57-year-old bank executive who prided herself on her exemplary active life outside of her desk job. Her grown children had moved on and she and her husband enjoyed life together. Mrs. E.J. had had her annual checkup three months earlier; she had passed with flying colours, but she had called her family doctor for an appointment because she had noted increasing shortness of breath when she was on the treadmill, which was unusual for her. She was scheduled to meet her doctor in a week. She was on no medications, and she was not a smoker but enjoyed a daily glass of wine. Following dinner one night, Mrs. J. was at the sink when she suddenly dropped a dish she was holding in her right hand. Her husband came to her side and asked her what was wrong, but Mrs. J. could not answer, and when she tried to walk out of the kitchen, it was clear that she was dragging her right leg. Her husband helped her to the sofa and laid her down. As soon as she was comfortable, he rushed to the telephone and dialed 911. The ambulance arrived in 12 minutes and the paramedics performed the FAST assessment shown in Figure 4. Based on Mrs. J.'s responses to FAST, the paramedics

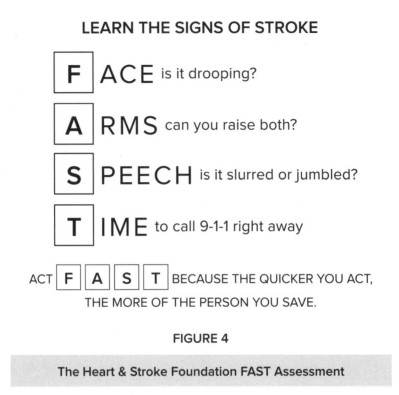

LEARN THE SIGNS OF STROKE

F ACE is it drooping?

A RMS can you raise both?

S PEECH is it slurred or jumbled?

T IME to call 9-1-1 right away

ACT **F** **A** **S** **T** BECAUSE THE QUICKER YOU ACT, THE MORE OF THE PERSON YOU SAVE.

FIGURE 4

The Heart & Stroke Foundation FAST Assessment

concluded she had suffered a stroke. They told her husband that her pulse was irregular, bundled her up, and drove her, sirens blaring, to the hospital designated as a stroke centre. From the ambulance, they called the emergency room and the hospital's locating clerk, who alerted the radiology department and the neurologist on call that the ambulance was bringing a patient suspected of suffering a stroke. On arriving at the ER, the patient's vital signs were taken and the signs of stroke were confirmed. Listening to her heart, the ER doctor suspected that she suffered from atrial fibrillation, which implied that the stroke may have been due to a blood clot that had formed in the heart because of this irregular rhythm, had dislodged, and gone to the left middle cerebral artery, which feeds the speech centre and the motor strip controlling the opposite arm.

The patient was whisked to the CT scanner, where it was confirmed that she had suffered a stroke and not a brain hemorrhage; the presence of a blood clot blocking the left middle cerebral artery was also ascertained. A drug called tissue plasminogen activator (tPA) was started intravenously to break up the clot, and simultaneously a catheter was introduced into her arterial supply, threaded all the way to the clot, which was then snared and pulled out. Mrs. J. immediately responded by being able to speak and answer questions appropriately. The speed of action and the availability of effective therapy had converted Mrs. J.'s stroke from lifelong misery to a passing illness.

The whole process, from onset of trouble and the husband calling 911 to the patient regaining her speech, had taken 90 minutes. During that time the brain region deprived of its blood supply was "holding its breath," causing symptoms, but the cells within the affected region were still alive, albeit on strike. The resumption of blood flow to the affected region resulted in immediate regaining of function. The time lapse from the sudden onset of trouble to the administration of tPA, 90 minutes, was well within the 3.5-hour limit from onset of stroke to treatment that is recommended.

Mrs. J. was able to walk out of the hospital in three days. She had fully regained her speech. She was also seen by a cardiologist, who prescribed a drug that would prevent the formation of blood clots, and she was given an appointment to treat her atrial fibrillation.

Not every stroke patient fares as well as Mrs. E.J. Neurology books describe a stroke as "lightning out of a blue sky." A stroke can occur when you least expect it and often without prior warning. Regardless of the cause, the sudden interruption

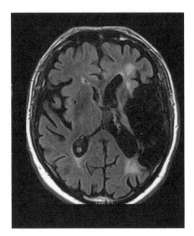

FIGURE 5

MRI scan of a patient who has suffered a
stroke that was not immediately treated

of blood supply to a sufficiently large area of the brain will usually result in immediate symptoms that the individual feels: sudden interruption of speech production or comprehension, sudden motor deficits such as weakness in an arm or dragging of one leg, a sudden severe headache, sudden loss of the ability to see out of one eye or partially from both eyes. If nothing is done rapidly to correct this situation, these deficits will become longstanding, until the rehabilitation and hard work of the patient at recovery gives back some of the functions he or she lost.

The image in Figure 5 shows what a major stroke on the patient's left half of the brain (on your right) looks like on MRI scan. It is that large dark spot in the middle right side of the image, often referred to as an infarct. That entire dark region used to contain brain, as on the normal side, but after it died the affected tissue was removed by the body's mechanisms that clean up debris and was then filled with cerebrospinal fluid

(CSF). This patient likely cannot speak, cannot understand what is being said, and is paralyzed on the right side of the body.

If you suddenly realize you can't do something you could do just a minute ago, you should assume you are suffering a stroke and immediately call 911 for an ambulance. Ideally, it will take you to an emergency room that has rapid access to brain imaging and trained personnel who can treat the stroke. Canadian Stroke Network scientists and clinicians recommend that no more than one hour be spent from the moment the stroke patient arrives at the hospital to when tPA is administered.

If the stroke is not treated in a timely fashion and damage to the brain occurs, cognitive impairment is likely to result. Many studies confirm that strokes are a major cause of impaired cognitive functions, including dementia. In one study, 57% of patients who suffered a stroke while they were free of any dementia developed some degree of cognitive trouble within the first year after the stroke. An additional 32.4% developed the lesser condition of MCI.[4] Thus a stroke will diminish, to a lesser or greater extent, the ability to think, remember, and make judgements in 90% of those unfortunate individuals who suffer this event and do not receive timely treatment.

The Sneaky Strokes You May Not Be Aware Of

There is a very important new category of brain-damaging events that can lead to dementia. It turns out that not all blockages of blood vessels in the brain result in symptoms that the individual feels. It is possible that a blood vessel that becomes blocked is so small that the individual does not feel anything is wrong at the time, or may feel a temporary deficit from which he or she recovers rapidly. We began to see these brain "scars" on CT scans and MRI scans in patients who suffered from high blood pressure or other vascular risk factors, and there were mainly three types:

1. Lacunes or lacunar infarcts, which are usually between 3 and 20 mm in diameter and are seen on scans as holes in the deeper brain structures, particularly in an area called the basal ganglia.

2. Microbleeds, which are small (less than 5 mm) accumulations of blood in any brain location, including both grey and white matter.

3. White matter hyperintensities (WMH), which occur in the white matter of the brain. They result from failure of blood to flow through the tiny arteries called arterioles. These are the most prevalent form of small vessel disease affecting the brain.

Initially, we called these vascular events that the patient had not felt but which appeared on imaging "silent" strokes, but we now call them covert strokes, because there is nothing silent about them. A covert stroke does not mean that nothing bad happened. A small area of the brain, usually deep inside it where the fast-conducting myelinated white fibres are, was deprived of its blood supply and became damaged. It is important to remember: occlusion of even a single penetrating vessel can lead to cognitive deficits.[5]

People affected by a covert stroke may notice a decline in their ability to think clearly as a result of the occlusion of a single arteriole or even a single penetrating blood vessel, but if this happens again and again, the individual will suffer dementia.

CASE STUDY

Mr. R.T. came to my clinic referred by his family doctor. This 42-year-old man's main complaint was that he had recently felt that his brain was "in a fog." He worked in a small company and had become the go-to person for all computer-related issues. He enjoyed that role as he had taken several evening courses on computer literacy. He told me his colleagues had recently stopped bringing him their computer challenges and asking for his help, which they had done in the past. He took that as confirmation of his own sense that his thinking had become muddled.

Mr. T. gave me several other examples of why he thought he was not as sharp as he used to be. He was married and had two sons, 11 and 14 years old. He and his wife both worked. He had recently forgotten to attend a parent–teacher meeting even though he had committed to be there. He also commented on his increasing dependence on reminder notes. His wife had also asked him to seek medical attention because of his memory difficulties. The only medical problem Mr. T. knew of was that his family doctor had told him his blood pressure was too high and prescribed him some medication, but Mr. T. said he wasn't ready to take pills every day at his young age. He denied suffering any transient episodes of speech difficulty, weakness, or numbness.

When I examined Mr. T., he was clearly overweight. He weighed 240 pounds on a 5'10" frame. His waist circumference was 118 cm. His blood pressure at rest was 155/94 mmHg. His neurological examination was normal,

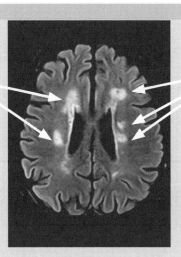

FIGURE 6

MRI scan of a patient who suffered covert strokes

The arrows point to white matter hyperintensities.

but he scored 24/30 on his MoCA test, confirming that indeed he had cognitive challenges.

I ordered an MRI scan and arranged to see him in four weeks. Figure 6 shows Mr. T.'s MRI scan.

The MRI showed that Mr. T. had suffered a number of covert small strokes, which left the scars evident in the white matter of his brain. The spots seen on the MRI and pointed out by the arrows represented areas of damage in the brain's white matter resulting from the blockage of small arteries. Other smaller areas of damage were also evident on this MRI. The MRI suggested that Mr. T. suffered from extensive small vessel disease in the brain. This likely explained why he complained of his brain being in a fog.

When Mr. T. returned four weeks later, I reviewed all the results with him, including showing him his MRI scan. I emphasized that his untreated high blood pressure was a significant risk to the health of his brain, and he seemed convinced of that. He asked me if there were ways to decrease his blood pressure that did not include taking daily medications. I told him that losing weight, becoming more active physically, and cutting down on salt would definitely help. I asked if whoever did the cooking at home added a lot of salt, and I was shocked at the answer: no one did any cooking at home. Mr. T. said he and his wife were too busy to go grocery shopping and cooking, so one of them brought home cooked food on a daily basis, frequently from fast food joints. The family had totally surrendered what it ate to third parties. This led to a much broader discussion about the need to consume fruits and vegetables, and to protect the future health of the family by emphasizing that time spent cooking was an investment in their future health rather than a waste of time.

Covert Strokes and Memory Function

One way to think of the deficit caused by small vessel disease is to think of the brain's white matter as the region where telephone lines coming from the neurons in the grey matter are coursing through. Interrupting these telephone lines means that the brain, which used to have rapid connections between site A and site B, now has to reroute the communication through site C. The connection will still occur, but it will be slow, require extra energy, and will be tedious. As a result, individuals who have suffered damage in their brains' white matter will process information more slowly and have difficulty with their memory. Thus covert strokes that result in damage to the fast-conducting myelinated white matter in the brain can not only impair memory function, but affect judgement and change personality.

Another way in which white-matter damage affects the brain is that it causes the brain's memory centre, the hippocampus, to shrink over time.[6] That process is called hippocampal sclerosis. Putting it all together, the conclusion is this: blockage in the brain's arterioles, which results in the WMHs we described earlier, affects cognitive and memory functions negatively.

What are the conditions associated with these small brain white-matter infarcts? Who is likely to get them? Dr. Sarah Vermeer in the Netherlands identified patients with small vessel disease in their brains and asked: "What else is wrong with them? What conditions or diseases could be associated with damage to the brain's white matter?[7] She reported that 43% of patients with high blood pressure (hypertension) showed small vessel disease in their brains, and 38% of patients with vascular risk factors such as diabetes and high cholesterol had the same finding. Surprisingly, 46% of patients who suffered from depression also showed these scars in their brains, confirming that sustained sadness affects brain structures negatively.

Vascular Disease and Alzheimer's Disease Influence Each Other

From what has been said so far, we can conclude that vascular disease is a major cause of dementia. Where does that leave

Alzheimer's disease? My colleague Dr. Sandy Black has studied the relationship between vascular disease and Alzheimer's disease, and her conclusions are very important. When the small blood vessels feeding the brain are not healthy, there are many consequences. In addition to interrupting brain circuits that are fed by the blocked arterioles or penetrating blood vessels, the fact that blood supply to that brain region is now reduced or interrupted means that the toxic proteins that are the hallmark of Alzheimer's disease, tau and β-amyloid, cannot be washed away rapidly, so they build up, causing the brain to suffer from their toxic effects.[8] Studies had shown some time ago that blood vessel blockages worsened Alzheimer's pathology.[9] After a recent review of the entire field was completed,[10] the consensus opinion is that vascular disease of the brain encourages Alzheimer's disease to flourish and eggs it on, and Alzheimer's disease proteins are toxic to brain cells and blood vessels. The combination becomes a very nasty state of affairs for the brain.

There is obviously a lot about this process that we still don't understand. If you are a carrier of the Alzheimer gene, your brain may be producing more of the toxic proteins associated with the condition, but what is very clear now to everyone is that vascular disease of the brain is a major driver of dementia. The good news is that while genetically inherited Alzheimer's disease and its consequences are not preventable or treatable, vascular disease of the brain is both preventable and treatable. This is the key to the assertion made in this book that we can control how well we age, and that dementia is not an unavoidable companion to aging. How, then, can we avoid getting vascular disease in the master organ? What are the risk factors that lead to blockages in the brain's blood vessels, small or large, resulting in overt and covert strokes?

Stroke Risk Factors

Figure 7 ranks the conditions that are associated with a high degree of risk for the development of vascular disease of the brain resulting in strokes, and their frequent consequence of dementia.[11]

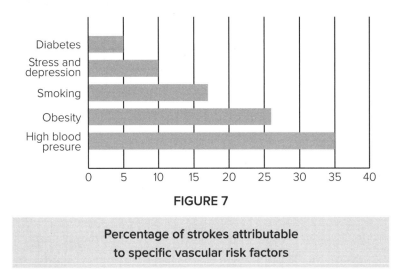

FIGURE 7

Percentage of strokes attributable to specific vascular risk factors

You can see from this figure that a number of conditions significantly increase the risk for a stroke to occur. The biggest risk factor is high blood pressure, causing 35% of all strokes. Other risk factors that are amenable to medical therapies include high cholesterol levels, diabetes, and a variety of cardiac disorders such as atrial fibrillation. Other vascular risk factors that increase the likelihood of suffering a stroke fit in a category we can call "lifestyle," and all of them can be controlled. Thus interventions that correct high blood pressure, integrating more physical activity into our daily lives, losing the excess weight, and mitigating some of the other lifestyle issues would substantially reduce our risk for stroke and its major consequence, dementia.

This figure emphasizes the point made by Dr. Gustavo Roman, a professor of neurology and specialist in Alzheimer's disease, and his colleagues. He states that "in community dwellings of the elderly, the most common forms of dementia involve the cerebral microvasculature."[12] He has found that practising clinicians can reasonably advise patients that "the management and treatment of vascular disease risk factors are likely beneficial not only to prevent heart disease and stroke, but also common forms of dementia in the community."

Can I Predict My Risk for Dementia?

A number of studies have found that it's possible to predict the likelihood of suffering dementia, but these prediction models apply only to populations, not to individuals. So although we can't predict an individual's risk for dementia, the associations that have been reported are nonetheless very instructive.

Researchers in Sweden have come up with a risk score for the prediction of dementia.[13] They evaluated individuals in midlife for risk factors associated with dementia and re-examined them 20 years later for signs of the condition. Their work resulted in a method to determine the probability of dementia in late life based on midlife risk scores (Table 1). To use the information in the table, find the score that applies to you, for each risk factor you have. Add up the scores. Remember that this information is not designed to give one individual's risk for dementia, but the total score is instructive nonetheless.

If the total score for a group of people is less than five, their chances of developing dementia in 20 years is low—the same as the general population with the same age. A total score of 6 or 7 almost doubles the risk, and if it climbs to 12 or more,

TABLE 1

Dementia risk in 20 years, based on scores for risk factors in midlife	
SCORING SYSTEM AND RISK OF LATE-ONSET DEMENTIA	
RISK FACTOR	**SCORE**
Age (Year)	
< 47	0
47–53	3
> 53	4
Education (Years)	
≥ 10	0
7–9	2
< 6	3
Systolic Blood Pressure (mm Hg)	
≤ 140	0
> 140	2
Body Mass Index (kg/m2)	
≤ 30	0
> 30	2
Total Cholesterol (mmol/L)	
≤ 6.5	0
> 6.5	2
Physical Activity	
Active	0
Inactive	1

the risk of dementia is 16 times that of a group that does not have those risk factors. As you can see, future dementia is significantly predicted by older age, low education (less than 10 years of school), high blood pressure, obesity, and high cholesterol.

This information was further refined in an important study published in 2011 by a professor of psychiatry and her colleagues.[14] It revealed the factors that contribute to dementia worldwide, but additionally assessed the contribution of each risk factor to dementia in North America. The relevant table from their article is shown in Table 2. Let's just look at education for a moment. The table reveals that low education may explain 19.1% of dementia worldwide but only 7.3% in North America. This is likely because early school education is more prevalent in North America than in poorer countries, and the brain is forced during the process of learning to create and sustain the internal connections among its various cells early in life. That constitutes building up of cognitive reserve. Later on in life, these early connections protect the brain from the influences that diminish or disrupt the thinking process.

TABLE 2

Factors contributing to dementia worldwide and in North America		
FACTOR	WORLDWIDE PROBABLE % ATTRIBUTION TO FACTOR	NORTH AMERICA PROBABLE % ATTRIBUTION TO FACTOR
Low education	19.1	7.3
Smoking	13.9	10.8
Physical inactivity	12.7	21.0
Depression	10.6	14.7
Hypertension	5.1	8.0
Diabetes	2.4	3.3
Obesity	2.0	7.3

When we explore the influence of education on the health of our minds, additional evidence comes to us from individuals who speak more than one language. If you have struggled to learn more than one language, your possibility of dementia is delayed.[15] When compared with those who speak only one language, those who commonly use two languages had a seven-fold increase in protection against cognitive impairment. The benefit of bilingualism to the brains and minds of individuals was again reviewed and confirmed recently.[16] There is one catch, however, to this benefit, and that is that you have to keep using both languages if you want to continue deriving the cognitive benefit. The brain is the ultimate capitalist: if you don't need it, if you don't use it, the brain won't waste energy maintaining the connections, and they will be lost. Remember: Use it or lose it! This study implies that our brains need to be stimulated intellectually, preferably at an early age but definitely at every period of life, and the stimuli need to be varied if we are to remain cognitively sharp.

The other factors in the table are topics discussed in this book and are the basis for some of the rules suggested to help us keep our marbles. In societies where some of these rules are part of their life, the rate of dementia is low. It may be hard for people in North America to accept this, but in societies with lower economic status, where life is not as sedentary as it is in rich societies, where the food is not as packed with empty calories, and where people are more likely to be socially connected because they have time on their hands and their hands are not busy with electronic gadgets, there is a lower incidence of dementia. I hope it is as striking to you as it was to me that physical inactivity contributes to 21% of the dementias in North America, but only 12% in the rest of the world.

The important point is this: We have the tools we need to shield our brains against dementia. You can keep your marbles if you make that an important goal for yourself, starting as early as possible, while remembering that it is never too late.

Vascular Supply to the Brain

To better understand the conditions that affect and weaken the brain's blood supply, let's examine the way blood is normally delivered to every brain cell, and then explore what happens when blood vessels feeding these brain cells are damaged.

The heart receives blood that has been loaded with oxygen as it coursed through the lungs. The heart pumps the blood out to provide energy to every organ in the body. The major artery that carries blood out of the heart is called the ascending aorta. As it gets close to the neck, it forms an arch so that it can begin its descent towards the lower part of the body. Blood vessels arise from this arch to supply the brain with the blood and energy it needs. There are essentially three major blood vessels that feed the brain. A vertebral artery courses through the vertebrae on either side of the back of your neck and join together to form a single artery called the basilar. The basilar artery feeds the brain stem and the back side of the brain. The other vessels supplying the brain are the two common carotid arteries, each going along one side of your neck to enter the skull and supply the rest of the brain. These carotid arteries branch into the external carotid artery that supplies your face and scalp and tongue with energy, and the internal carotid artery that goes to the brain. Inside the brain this artery branches further into a number of smaller arteries that course along the surface of the brain and other smaller ones that penetrate into the brain, providing every last brain cell with the energy it needs. Each artery on the brain's surface now does what the city has to do to bring water into household taps from the main water lines: it breaks itself up into smaller and smaller arteries, and we go from arteries to arterioles, which now penetrate into the brain then break down further into penetrating tiny blood vessels called microvessels. This way, every one of the billions of cells in the brain receives the blood it needs. The larger arteries supply the grey mantle of the brain where the neurons are concentrated, and the arterioles and penetrating microvessels supply blood to the white matter of the brain.

The description of the brain's arterial and venous architecture shows that your brain is exquisitely dependent on its blood supply. This organ that does not move, pump, or contract, and that weighs only 1.4 kg, consumes almost 30% of the energy available for the entire body. The blood vessels that bring this energy to the brain are designed to maintain this energy supply. For instance, a phenomenon called autoregulation allows the blood vessels feeding the brain to dilate or constrict to maintain a relatively constant blood flow to the brain while you are going about your daily activities. Whether you are sitting, walking, running, thinking, or conversing, the brain's energy requirements are met under all circumstances through the response of the blood vessels feeding it. During your normal daily life, your brain's blood supply is flexible and satisfies any energy call you make on your brain.

What Happens in the Brain While the Patient Is Suffering a Stroke?

The brain is an energy pig! Under normal circumstances, every minute, 55 mL of blood bathe every 100 g of brain. When an artery supplying the brain begins to narrow, either due to atherosclerosis or because a blood clot affected a brain region's blood supply, the flow of blood gets reduced. But the individual might not be aware of any consequences because the system is over-designed to protect the brain. As blood flow falls below the normal 55 mL/100 gm/min, the brain continues to function normally all the way down to 20 mL/100 gm/min. It does this by extracting more oxygen and glucose from the remaining trickle of blood. The patient is able to walk, talk, think, and remember completely normally despite a 63% reduction in the flow of blood to the affected region of the brain.

Below this level of flow, when flow to 100 g of brain gets below 20 mL/min, brain cells cannot function normally, but they will stay alive for a short few hours—three or four. In the case of Mrs. J., it was the left part of her brain that was "holding its breath," resulting in speech difficulty and right-sided weakness. If during this critical period of time, blood flow returns to above 20 mL/100 gm/min, say because the clot broke up and moved on, the symptoms will disappear and function will return to normal. Mrs. J.'s blood flow to her brain returned to normal because she received ideal medical care by going to an emergency room that was set up to deal with strokes. Permanent damage to the brain will result only if blood flow remains below this critical level for more than three to four hours. Brain cells will survive below that level for a time determined by how low the flow is: death of brain cells is instantaneous below the level of 12 mL/100 gm/min; between 20 and 12 mL, cell survival depends on the level of blood flow remaining.

Transient, or Threatened, Strokes

What if a person experiences the sudden onset of symptoms, like weakness in an arm or loss of speech function, but the symptoms resolve and the person affected feels completely back to normal, say, in 20 minutes? That is called a transient ischemic attack (TIA), and it usually implies that the deficit occurred because a blood clot travelled to the brain and blocked a blood vessel feeding the part of brain that, as a consequence, stopped working, resulting in the symptoms. The patient's symptoms disappeared likely because the clot eventually broke up in response to the body's natural defence mechanisms and blood flow was restored to the affected part of the brain within minutes. While this individual should be congratulated for avoiding a brain-damaging stroke, he or she is at risk for a major one and should immediately seek medical attention to find out the cause of the TIA and take the necessary measures to prevent a big stroke from occurring. A stroke can often occur in the 24 hours that follow a TIA, so it is extremely urgent and important to attend to it. The other important point about TIAs is that even though they are transient deprivations of the brain's blood supply, the brain does not forgive the insult, and individuals who have suffered TIAs often run the risk of having some cognitive trouble even if they never suffered a completed stroke.[17] A TIA is an emergency and should be attended to immediately.

The Brain Is Able to Repair Itself

If you went to your doctor complaining of memory difficulty and investigations revealed that you had suffered covert strokes, should you give up hope of regaining the lost function? Not at all. Injury to the brain, such as from a stroke, whether overt or covert, leads to the mobilization of all available brain-repair mechanisms to try to circumvent the deficit. This should give us all reason to hope that deficits sustained by stroke can be reduced and may even be completely overcome.

When damage occurs, the brain assigns the job that the injured brain area used to do, such as speaking or moving an arm, to new brain areas. These secondary brain regions are not as capable or as fast as the original, but their efficiency and ultimate success are very dependent on the messages we send the brain through our actions. For instance, if a stroke results in paralysis of the left arm, the natural impulse is to ignore the left arm and simply use the right arm. That hampers the recovery process because the brain does not receive the message that you want to improve the function of the left arm. If you don't instruct your brain by attempting to use the weak arm, it will not waste energy doing something you may not want or need it to do. Understanding this phenomenon has led to a form of therapy for post-stroke recovery called constraint-induced therapy. Essentially, the good arm, in this case the right, is put in a sling to prevent it from being used, so that the patient is forced to use the paralyzed arm. The message sent to the brain is "Yes, I want to improve the function of my weak left arm. Get on with it. Do what you have to do. I am telling you what I want."

In the fetus, stem cells are in full action forming the brain in all its structural complexity. Normal stem cell action in the fetal brain is essential for subsequent normal cognition. Stem cells do not disappear at the moment of birth. On the contrary, they are there even in the adult brain in storage sites ready to get to work. When an injury occurs, stem cells are mobilized from their storage sites to attempt to get to the injury region, metamorphose themselves into new brain cells, and learn to do the job of the injured and dead cells. And as we have said, one stem cell storage site is entirely dedicated to serving the memory centre in our brain, the hippocampus. Many of the actions and lifestyles I recommend to improve memory lead to the mobilization of these stem cells so that the hippocampus is constantly refreshed, new memories can be easily formed, and old ones can be easily recalled. As you will see later, individuals who are physically active have larger hippocampi on brain scans and have far better preserved memory functions than those who are sedentary, because physical activity is one very important mechanism to mobilize stem cells that serve memory functions.

This even works after damage to the brain has occurred through vascular disease and cognitive ability is reduced. Mr. T. asked me what recovery he could hope for, and he was motivated. He knew that his career and his family's well-being depended on his recovery. He made a complete turnaround in his lifestyle and doggedly pursued a better diet for himself and his family, resulting in weight loss and a reduction in his hypertension. He attended a program where practical memory-improving strategies were taught. He was also motivated to learn ways of reducing his stress through exercise. After six months, he could not give up exercising because it had improved his mood, his cognitive ability, his efficiency and productivity at work, and he had learned the value of socializing away from his TV. He was an individual confirmation of the results of a study led by my colleague Dr. Brad McIntosh, who showed that regular exercise improved the ability of brain centres important for memory and thinking efficiency to talk to each other.[18]

The Genetics of Alzheimer's Disease

We suspect that a patient suffering from dementia has Alzheimer's disease as the predominant cause if:

1. The age of onset of the cognitive and thinking difficulties is in the 40s or early 50s;

2. More than 10 to 15% of the members of the patient's family suffer from dementia; and

3. All other risk factors that may negatively affect the blood vessels in the brain have been eliminated.

A person under the age of 50 showing cognitive difficulty and memory trouble may well be suffering from the genetic variety of Alzheimer's disease, particularly if there are other members of the family also affected by dementia. Although such individuals represent less than 2% of dementia cases, it is important to recognize them and, if they are willing, test their blood relatives to see if they have inherited the disease. The reason for this is that an individual has to receive only one copy of the gene to show the disease, meaning that the inheritance is autosomal dominant. So let's take a quick look at the genetics of Alzheimer's disease.

When a young person, say 45 years old, begins to show memory and behaviour difficulties that progress to dementia, with brain scans suggesting loss of brain mass and atrophy, genetic testing may reveal a genetic predisposition to Alzheimer's disease. That means the individual may have inherited one or more genes that carry the code for making the toxic β-amyloid and tau proteins we talked about. Three genes have been identified that can promote the formation of these proteins. They are called the β-amyloid precursor protein gene and the presenelin1 and presenelin2 genes. About half of the young patients who develop dementia of the Alzheimer type have mutations in one or more of these genes, which results in the excessive accumulation of β-amyloid, the primary driver of Alzheimer's disease pathology. This is what leads to the formation of the plaques and tangles discussed earlier.

When dementia occurs after the age of 65, the genetic mutations in these three genes are thought to play a minor role. Although these individuals may have a genetic variant that slows down the brain's ability to rid itself of β-amyloid, called the Apo E gene, genetic testing to identify this gene abnormality is reserved for people who develop dementia under the age of 45. For most cases of late-onset dementia, it is generally agreed that vascular disease of the brain, lifestyle, and environment play a major role in its appearance.

Why Alzheimer's disease without any vascular complications leads to dementia is still a matter of some debate. A number of hypotheses or theories have evolved, the main ones arising from the observations referred to earlier, namely the accumulation of β-amyloid and tau proteins. The hypothesis is that deposits of β-amyloid protein are toxic to brain cells. This protein is produced as a result of the activity of a gene located on chromosome 21, and support for this hypothesis came partly from the knowledge that patients with trisomy 21 (Down's syndrome), who have an extra gene copy of chromosome 21, almost universally show the signs of Alzheimer's disease as they get older. The tau hypothesis states that the strands that accumulate inside the nerve cells cause damage to the vital structures within the cell, making it impossible for the cell to get rid of toxins that accumulate during normal neuronal activity. The tangles eventually lead to the death of the cells. Unfortunately, to date we have no effective treatments against Alzheimer's disease. Attempts to develop pharmacological treatments that have focused on eliminating the β-amyloid deposits have failed, and a vaccine that cleared this protein from the brain also had no significant impact on the dementia.

In the general population, more than 95% of patients develop dementia after the age of 65, and this book's central premise is that in that setting, vascular health, lifestyle, and environment play determining roles in the clinical expression of the disease. Harmful lifestyle and environmental conditions affect the blood supply to the brain and can lead to vascular disease that threatens the brain's integrity. Thus even if genetic testing of older patients with dementia confirms the presence of mutations associated with Alzheimer's disease, all is not lost, and following the rules in this book, as was evident in the Nun Study and other aging studies, will improve the chances of keeping dementia at bay.

It is important to remember that genes aren't the be all and end all. Genes can be turned on or off by what is now called epigenetic factors, and these are known to be substantially influenced by the physical, emotional, and social environments of the individual as well as his or her behaviour. Scientists learned a long time ago that genes are not the only factors that determine whether you get a condition or you don't. What matters is what you do with the genes you inherited. The important point is this: genes are only guideposts for both our physical and mental health, but their function is influenced by other factors we can control. Consequently, genetic testing is not recommended for patients who develop dementia late in their lives, but it is recommended in early-onset dementia. While that may determine the likelihood that the progeny of a person with early-onset disease will also be affected, little can be offered to help those who are diagnosed with pure Alzheimer's disease. A recent study concluded that drugs currently used to treat dementia did not in fact improve function among patients suffering from milder forms of cognitive impairment.[19] As a result, there is much less enthusiasm to try new medications against Alzheimer's disease.

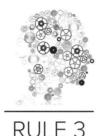

RULE 3

Monitor and Tame Your Blood Pressure

Let's start this rule by going to the pathology lab to look at blood vessels. As we have learned, the three major types of blood vessels in the body are arteries, veins, and arterioles.

A normal large blood vessel is an artery that is 3 cm across. It has an inner lining of glistening smooth tissue that is in direct contact with the blood flowing through. If you strip this smooth layer off, you come to a layer made of elastic tissue that allows the blood vessel to constrict or dilate. If you poke it, it feels like pushing on a rubber band. Just below this layer is a more meaty-looking layer of tissue. If you touch it, it feels like fibre, and this layer is bound on the outside by another layer of elastic tissue.

This is the layering arrangement in a large artery that carries blood out of the heart to major organs like the lungs, kidneys, and brain. As the artery gets closer to the organ it is supplying, it branches into smaller arteries that have the same layering arrangement. This type of artery, however, doesn't go into the organ it is supplying. That job is left to arterioles, the smaller arteries that are perhaps 2 mm in diameter or smaller. The arterioles are the final direct feeders of all our organs, including the brain. In fact, the big arteries themselves are supplied by arterioles because, as living hard-working tissue, they need to be nourished too.

We have arteries, small and large, that we can examine in a patient who died after a massive stroke. The carotid artery of such a patient looks very different from the normal one. The smooth glistening inner layer in the normal artery described earlier is anything but smooth and glistening in this patient. The layer is raised into the vessel's opening. It feels rough, and instead of having a healthy pink look, it has a yellow-brown, discoloured look, and the entire length of the artery is similarly changed. In fact, this patient's stroke was due to the carotid artery becoming blocked with these fatty protrusions into the space where the blood flows. We call this atherosclerosis. When atherosclerosis is extensive, it narrows the opening of the blood vessel and the flow of blood to the brain can diminish below the brain's needs, causing a stroke.

This patient had vascular disease, and as we have learned, vascular disease is the major cause of dementia. And the biggest risk factor for vascular disease is hypertension, or high blood pressure. In this chapter we will learn what constitutes high blood pressure, how to measure it properly, and what the consequences of high blood pressure can be. Fortunately, blood pressure can be measured painlessly and at minimal or no cost, and can be managed easily.

Your blood pressure is composed of two simple numbers that are packed with information about your health. The higher number is called the systolic pressure and indicates what the peak pressure inside your arteries is when the heart has just contracted, sending blood rushing up and down the blood vessels, putting "pressure" on their walls. The lower number, which is called the diastolic pressure, is the pressure within your arteries when the blood vessels are relaxed. So the numbers tell us a lot about your heart function, the stress on your blood vessels, and their ability to relax.

In this chapter I will define a healthy BP range and the actions that are necessary to bring your blood pressure to that healthy range if and when it is elevated. Let me not mince words: maintaining your blood pressure in the normal range is your best guarantee against dementia.

The Consequences of High Blood Pressure

When blood pressure is too high, one possible and greatly feared consequence is that a blood vessel inside the brain will burst, resulting in a brain hemorrhage. If that outcome is avoided but blood pressure remains at an elevated level, the blood vessels thicken their walls to protect themselves against bursting! That is what we call hardening of the arteries or atherosclerosis. This unfortunate process is accelerated when we spend too much time being inactive. The arteries also stiffen up in the setting of diabetes, high cholesterol, and too much fat in the blood, as well as in individuals who smoke or drink excessively. The hardening of the arteries in turn narrows the space available for the blood to flow through, requiring the heart to pump harder and raising the pressure in the blood vessels. As you might guess, if the process of wall thickening continues, the heart pumps harder and harder and may become exhausted and suffer damage. The blood vessels may eventually get clogged up, and when the brain is the affected organ, that can cause strokes, as we saw in the earlier example.

Higher than normal blood pressure is not only an indication that your blood vessels are unhealthy, but it is also a harbinger of trouble to come. It is estimated that two-thirds of strokes are due to uncontrolled high blood pressure. High blood pressure, if untreated and persistent, will put your vascular system into a vicious cycle: elevated blood pressure will lead to damage to many organs, including the brain, the heart, the kidneys, and the retina of the eyes. This in turn will cause a further elevation in blood pressure as these damaged organs demand blood at a higher pressure to function properly. This will then lead to a higher elevation in blood pressure and more damage occurring in these same body organs. Consequently, individuals with high blood pressure (hypertension) are four times more likely to die of stroke as people with normal blood pressure. The brain is the favourite target organ when blood pressure is sustained at a higher than normal level, but it is important to stress that individuals with hypertension are also likely to suffer heart disease, kidney failure needing dialysis, and retinal degeneration leading to blindness.

And what about the impact of high blood pressure on our cognitive functions, our ability to remember and to make sound judgements? The relationship of dementia to high blood pressure is very straightforward. If a group of individuals had their blood pressure measured in their 50s, and they were tested for their cognitive ability with thinking and memory tests some 25 years later, the result would be stated as follows: Every 1 mmHg in systolic blood pressure sustained above 110 mmHg increases the likelihood of dementia in later life by 1% (recall that blood pressure is measured in millimetres of mercury, which has the symbol Hg).

Elevated blood pressure has been associated with the occurrence of large strokes, lacunar infarcts, microinfarcts, and diffuse white matter hyperintensities. So it is *extremely* important to maintain blood pressure in the normal range. And don't wait till you are advanced in age to control your blood pressure: the fact that blood pressure in the middle years is the determinant of brain health in later years was recently confirmed by a large study.[2] It is crucial, for the health of your brain, to keep blood pressure normal.

Causes of High Blood Pressure

Our blood pressure generally increases with age. As we get older, our blood vessels become a little stiffer, and so for the same volume of blood, the increased arterial stiffness will cause the pressure against the walls of the blood vessels to go higher. So any condition that will (a) thicken the walls and increase the stiffness of the blood vessels, (b) increase the volume of their contents, or (c) squeeze the blood vessels from outside will increase blood pressure, leading to the grave consequences we have outlined.

Specifically then, in addition to getting older or having inherited a predisposition to high blood pressure, the main potentially modifiable conditions that will lead to hypertension are these:

1. **Excess salt** in our diet is a major driver of high blood pressure. We know what excess salt does to us: it tightens the blood vessels and increases the resistance to the flow of blood, resulting in hypertension. We don't know all the different ways by which salt brings this about, but we know that when we consume too much salt, the

brain senses this and increases activity of the sympathetic system, which triggers constriction of the blood vessels. Also, eating too much salt makes us thirsty so we tend to drink more, perhaps water but perhaps also high-calorie drinks that make us put on weight, resulting in a higher volume of blood and high blood pressure. The Canadian Stroke Network recommends a daily intake of 1500 mg or less of sodium—that is less than 4 g or ¾ of a teaspoonful of salt for the day.

2. The **sugar** that we consume when we drink too many beverages, eat too much cereal or too many cakes, biscuits, or muffins increases our blood pressure because it interacts with the lining of our blood vessels and makes them tighten up. The recommendation of the World Health Organization is that an adult should not exceed an intake of 50 g (1.7 oz) of sugar per day, and half of that would be even better.[3] When you consider that a 355 mL bottle of soft drink may contain 35 g of sugar, you can see that the limit is quite stringent and leaves no room for consuming large bottles of soft drinks. Importantly, sugar in fresh fruit is exempted from this limit.

3. **Obesity** is a growing problem in Western societies and a major driver of dementia. Think of the excess fat as not only squeezing the major blood vessels in the body and raising blood pressure, but also a factory producing nasty chemicals. I have devoted the next chapter to this problem.

4. **Smoking** does contribute to hypertension, so think of cigarettes this way. With every puff of smoke you take, your blood turns a little less red and a little more blue, depriving your brain of the energy it needs to function properly. With every puff inhaled, the smoker introduces

more toxins into the body and makes the lining of the blood vessels feeding the brain more inflamed and angry. Smokers also get more diabetes. All of that will worsen brain function, so smoking has been recognized as a risk factor for dementia.[4] Smokers have a 45% greater risk of developing dementia than non-smokers. I do not want to minimize how difficult it is to quit smoking—it is one of the most addictive habits on this earth—but many have succeeded in quitting smoking, and you can too.

I remember stepping out the door at the Montreal Neurological Institute and coming across one of the orderlies I knew. He had come out to smoke. I stopped and chatted, and he admitted he had tried many times to stop smoking and had failed. When he had finished smoking, I took him up to my lab and showed him pictures of lungs obtained at autopsy from smokers and non-smokers. He never smoked again. The horrible pictures on cigarette boxes, the increased taxes, and the fact that smokers have come under social pressure have proven their value— we need to take similar measures with other recognized health risks.

Stories like this make an important point about quitting smoking: it is essential to have a reason to do it. The reason provides the energy to quit, admittedly a very difficult activity. That is not a sufficient condition, however. It helps to have people around you who support you and will remind you on days when you might falter that no, you don't need a cigarette.

5. Excessive and persistent **alcohol** intake can lead to dementia. The medical literature suggests that "excessive drinking" can be defined as anything more than two glasses of wine

per day or their equivalent, which is somewhere around 300 mL of wine per day. There are in fact suggestions that low levels of alcohol intake protect the brain against dementia, but this has not been conclusively proven. We do know that persistent intake of alcohol above that level will raise blood pressure. People who have more than two drinks a day are twice as likely to have hypertension as those who abstain, and both heavy drinking and binge drinking will increase the tendency to form blood clots and to suffer bleeds into the brain. Another major impact of high alcohol intake is poor nutrition, resulting in thiamine deficiency, which as we saw can cause severe short-term memory deficits. Put together, 80% of individuals who consume excessive and persistent amounts of alcohol will sustain some damage to their brains.[5]

6. A **sedentary lifestyle** may be increasingly imposed on us by modern life's demands and the wired world. We sit a lot, and as we will see in Rule 5, a sedentary lifestyle is associated with raised blood pressure and results in weaker memory and cognitive functions.

7. Insufficient or **poor-quality sleep** will contribute to hypertension. Sleeping long enough to feel rested is not a luxury. It is the opportunity for the brain to rejuvenate itself and for our blood vessels to relax. This is so important that I have devoted the entire Rule 6 to this issue.

8. We have known for a while that **persistent loneliness, high anxiety, and depression** have major negative impacts on our blood vessels and lead to raised blood pressure.[6] These conditions can impair our mind. I have devoted Rule 7 to this important driver of dementia and how to avoid it.

9. There is growing evidence that persistent **exposure to air pollution** will weaken cognitive functions partly through its impact on atherosclerosis. Studies were performed in London, England, and in Boston, and the results are concordant: residential proximity to a major roadway will lead to declining performance on cognitive tests, including verbal learning and memory as well as executive functioning.[7,8]

10. **Noise**, if not pleasant to our ears, raises our blood pressure and impairs our memory functions. Exposure to occupational noise, particularly at levels above 85 decibels, significantly increases the likelihood of hypertension.[9] In contrast, listening to music we like improves our reasoning ability. Unpleasant noise is always interpreted by our brain as a threat, and our body reacts to it by raising blood pressure and increasing tension to ready us to face the perceived threat. If this situation is chronic it will age our blood vessels and increase our chances of impairing our memory and other cognitive functions.

What Is Normal Blood Pressure?

The current definition of the blood pressure needed to maintain a healthy brain and mind is a systolic blood pressure equal to or less than 120 mmHg, and a diastolic blood pressure equal to or less than 80 mmHg. Having said that, science is still looking for precise answers to the question of what is a healthy systolic blood pressure, and the tendency clearly is to aim for systolic values that are lower than 130 mmHg, perhaps as low as 110 mmHg. A clinical trial run by NIH, called SPRINT (Systolic Blood Pressure Intervention Trial), compared outcomes, looking at heart attacks and strokes, when systolic blood pressure was maintained either below 140 mmHg or below 120 mmHg. The study showed such health advantages for the second group that the trial was stopped before it was supposed to because the answer was clear.[10] Importantly, the study population was diverse and included the elderly as well as women and ethnic and racial minorities. It is crucial to aim for a systolic blood pressure of 120 mm Hg or less when we are at rest.

Recently, when I was in a pharmacy, a woman sat down at the BP measuring station and took her own pressure. She took the printout with her pressure values to a pharmacy attendant for his interpretation. He looked at it and said to her, "You are okay. Anything under 160 is okay." I was dismayed so I followed her out of the store and approached her gently, informing her I was a physician, and explained to her that she should aim for the upper number in her BP reading to be at or below 120.

The medical literature is now very clear: resting blood pressure sustained at levels higher than 120 systolic increases the likelihood of stroke, and reducing blood pressure to this level or below reduces the likelihood of disease in the blood vessels feeding the brain. This information is not found in the advice on several websites about blood pressure. Indeed, even advice given by some health care providers often sets higher limits. There is still a range of blood pressure some refer to as "prehypertension," usually systolic blood pressure between 130 and 150 mmHg. The hope in coming up with this term was that someone whose blood pressure is in that range would take measures to reduce his or her blood pressure without medication, by making changes in diet and lifestyle that can reduce blood pressure. Unfortunately, that does not always work, and pretty soon both patient and health care provider move on to other things, leaving this major risk to the health of the brain unchecked. So no more dilly-dallying: aim for a resting systolic blood pressure of 120 mmHg or below.

The Problem of High Blood Pressure in Our Society

A large study was undertaken in 2013 in 17 countries across the spectrum of per-capita income; it revealed that more than 40% of the population had blood pressure above 140/90 mmHg. Awareness of hypertension and its treatment and control decline with lower income and less education.[11] A 2010 study by the National Center for Health Statistics conducted in American assisted-living facilities showed that 57% of the residents had high blood pressure, and a high percentage of them had suffered other consequences of vascular disease.[12] That is an astounding figure when you remember that high blood pressure is a treatable condition.

In Canada, the situation is not much better. Despite improvement in the control of hypertension over the past few years, thanks to the concerted efforts of Hypertension Canada and the Canadian Hypertension Education Program, a study by Statistics Canada in 2010 showed that one in five Canadians had systolic blood pressures above 140 mmHg, and an additional 20% had systolic blood pressure between 120 and 139 mmHg.[13] A more recent study in two mid-sized communities in Ontario showed that 41.4% of seniors had either untreated or uncontrolled hypertension.[14]

As if this was not bad enough, more worrisome is what is going on with our youth. A table published by Statistics Canada shows that over the ten years from 1994 to 2005 there was almost a tripling of the number of individuals between the ages of 12 and 34 who suffered from high blood pressure, and a doubling of high blood pressure in those between the ages of 35 and 39. I will explore some of the likely causes of this major setback to our public health, but it is worthwhile mentioning here one probable reason for this rise in blood pressure among young people: overall they are more sedentary than they used to be. It is estimated that young people, worldwide, spend on average more than eight hours a day being totally sedentary, which probably contributes to making them more obese than young people of previous generations.[15] Consequently, they are not as physically fit and not as fast as their elders used to be at their age.[16] For all these reasons, the World Health Organization identified high blood pressure as the leading risk factor for death and forecasted an epidemic of hypertension.

Measure and Record Your Blood Pressure

Do you know what your blood pressure at rest is? If not, then sadly you are in good company. A recent study in the United States showed that 76% of individuals whose blood pressure at rest was more than 140/90 mmHg were aware of this, 65% of them took treatment for it, but only 37% had resting blood pressure below this level.[17] This major killer and huge risk factor for dementia is easy to measure, painlessly and cheaply, but a lot of people don't know what their blood pressure is.

Individuals who measure their blood pressure at home often find it is higher when it is measured at the doctor's office. Blood pressure is designed to go up when the body demands more blood, such as when we exercise or are anxious, as we might be at the doctor's office. So it is important to measure blood pressure when we are relaxed and in familiar surroundings because resting blood pressure is the most significant number.

I recommend that my patients buy a BP measuring device to use at home. It is the best investment you will ever make for good health. Make sure you understand how to use it by asking the salesperson where you bought it, or a nurse or your physician. Every week, on the day of the week you are least likely to be stressed, sit down in a quiet spot, put the blood pressure cuff on, relax your legs and body for a minute or so, then take the pressure measurement. Write the top and bottom values down against the date of the measurement on a continuous record you keep. When you visit your doctor, take the record of these resting BP values with you to discuss them with her or him. If the blood pressure is consistently elevated, ask what you can do about it yourself, and if some of the measures suggested below do not reduce your blood pressure into the normal range, demand that something be done about it medically.

How to Lower Your Blood Pressure

Many of the causes of high blood pressure outlined earlier are preventable and manageable. Many organizations, including the Canadian Hypertension Society, the Heart and Stroke Foundation, and the Mayo Clinic, have outlined ways to reduce your blood pressure before medication is needed. Here is a list of the consensus advice. In the next chapters, I will give more detail about how to reduce blood pressure and consequent vascular disease.

1. Lose weight if you carry excess pounds: the closer you are to normal weight the more normal your blood pressure will be.

2. Modify your diet to reduce calories and sodium, and increase consumption of fruits, vegetables, and low-fat dairy products.

3. Limit your alcohol intake to two drinks or less per day.

4. Become more physically active.

5. Develop good sleep hygiene.

6. Increase social interaction and reduce stress.

7. If you are a smoker, quit.

Table 3 shows the effect of reductions in blood pressure, achieved without drugs and by making some of the recommended changes in your lifestyle.[18]

TABLE 3

Relative blood pressure effects of some major lifestyle modifications		
MODIFICATION	RECOMMENDATION	SYSTOLIC BLOOD PRESSURE REDUCTION
Reduce weight	Maintain BMI at 18.5–24.9	4.4 mmHg (for 5.1 kg weight loss)
Adopt DASH eating plan	Consume a diet rich in fruits, vegetables, and low-fat dairy products with a reduced content of saturated and total fat	5.5–11.4 mmHg (5.5 for normotensives, 11.4 for hypertensives)

continued...

TABLE 3

Relative blood pressure effects of some major lifestyle modifications		
MODIFICATION	RECOMMENDATION	SYSTOLIC BLOOD PRESSURE REDUCTION
Reduce dietary sodium	Reduce dietary sodium intake to no more than 2.4 g sodium (or 6 g of salt)	4–7 mmHg (for reduction by 6 g of daily salt intake)
Engage in physical activity	Engage in aerobic physical activity 30–60 min/day, 3–5 days/week	5 mmHg
Moderate alcohol consumption	Limit to no more than 2 drinks per day (men) or 1 drink per day (women)	3 mmHg (for 67% reduction from 3–6 drinks/day)

Obviously, if blood pressure can be brought down to normal levels through conservative means, that would be ideal; such reductions can be obtained with simple improvements in eating, drinking, and exercise habits. If that is not possible, however, you must talk to your physician about medical means of reducing blood pressure. There are many medications designed to reduce blood pressure, and many have little in the way of side effects. Your doctor might worry about reducing blood pressure too much, causing you to become dizzy when you stand up, with the potential for falls and consequent fractures. I don't wish that on anyone, but let us not hesitate to treat elevated blood pressure now that we know its potential ravages on the brain and the mind. If we must take medications to lower blood pressure to a systolic of 120 mmHg, let's do it, carefully, but do it we must.

Does Lowering Blood Pressure to Normal Decrease Dementia Risk?

The answer is an unequivocal yes. You have seen that decreasing the incidence of stroke will protect the brain from dementia. Decreasing the elevated systolic blood pressure by 10 mmHg will lower the likelihood of stroke by 38%, and if high blood pressure is lowered by 20 mmHg the likelihood of stroke will go down by 60%. So lowering blood pressure if the systolic value is above 120 mmHg will definitely make your brain more resistant to dementia. Some studies have been unable to show this benefit because they looked at cognition too soon after blood pressure was normalized, or used inadequate measures to assess cognition. However, as little as six months of treating high blood pressure has been beneficial to cognitive function.[19] This is not a new finding: a 1998 population-wide study showed that blood pressure management reduced brain atrophy in older individuals.[20] More recently, an analysis of data that included several trials demonstrated that treating high blood pressure even in the elderly had a protective effect on the ability to think and remember,[21] and a review of the literature confirms this conclusion.[22]

For this reason, we should celebrate recent successes in the management of blood pressure at the population level. Kaiser Permanente, a health care consortium in some U.S. states, has succeeded in increasing the percentage of patients whose hypertension is under control from 44% in 2001 to 87% in 2010.[23] They have also seen a decline in stroke mortality by

42% in those groups. In Canada, the latest data suggest that progress has also been made, but there is still a lot of room for improvement. For instance, in a study where blood pressure was measured in the general population, 32% of those with high blood pressure did not have it under control.[24]

Accomplishing Lifestyle Changes

Table 3 is very instructive. It was put together by the Canadian Hypertension Education Program from the medical literature available. You can see from this table that we could easily reduce blood pressure by modifying some of our eating, drinking, and other habits. Frequently, these issues are collectively referred to as "lifestyle," meaning that we have a measure of control on whether we indulge in them.

The challenge is that lifestyle changes are not easy to make. For one thing, there is rarely any follow-up by the health care system to encourage adherence to BP-lowering measures. Instead, in my experience, it is wishful thinking to simply suggest changes in lifestyle to individuals suffering from hypertension and expect it will happen. This is likely what explains the results of a recent health analysis issued by the U.S. Centers for Disease Control and Prevention showing that 67 million adult Americans had high blood pressure, but only 31 million of them had it treated appropriately. The remaining 36 million had high blood pressure that was untreated even though 88% of them got regular medical care. Our health care system, my colleagues the physicians, hospital administrators, and politicians need to be convinced that not managing elevated blood pressure in the millions of our citizens who suffer from hypertension will result in untold suffering for them and their families and cost the health care budgets billions.

Once your mind is absolutely made up to reduce your blood pressure into the normal range, you can increase the chances of success by sharing your goal with someone, ideally someone who cares about you. When a family member asks on a regular basis, by prior agreement, how you are coming along with this new challenge, it seems to encourage you to stick with the program. If your doctor's office calls you once in a while to ask how you are coming along in a smoking cessation program, it will increase your chances of success. Similarly, if a neighbour will go for regular walks with you, it's harder to get lazy and you have someone to share the challenge with. All these methods have been tried and proven to increase the likelihood of success.

I wish it was possible to include with your tax return a simple form signed by your doctor, where he or she indicates that your blood pressure on multiple readings throughout the previous year was normal, so that you would get a $25 break on your taxes. I'm sure this would significantly increase the attempt many of us make to normalize our blood pressure. There would be no difficulty showing the government that the resulting reduction in strokes, heart attacks, and cognitive decline would provide it with enormous returns on its investment. Some people are horrified at the idea that private medical information would be shared with a government agency. I get it, but I still believe it would be tremendously effective!

There is no room for complacency when it comes to managing our blood pressure. Look at it this way: What would you do if while you were driving at 60 miles an hour (110 km/hour) a message appeared on your dashboard that said: "Warning: your left wheel may come off at any time, but we recommend you continue driving calmly." I believe that reassuring someone with high blood pressure that they are in the prehypertension stage and should not worry about it is akin to saying "This high blood pressure is damaging your brain, but hey, relax."

Improving Cardiovascular Health at the Population Level

The authors of a 2011 study, which was given broad recognition and awarded many prizes, wanted to test the effectiveness of a community-based program modelled after the Cardiovascular Health Awareness Program (CHAP) and measure its impact, in a real-life setting, on diseases caused by vascular insufficiency such as heart attacks, stroke, and congestive heart failure.[25] The essential elements of CHAP were as follows: there was a community-wide orientation with a view to reaching all people in the community. Cardiovascular risk assessment sessions were offered free of charge and the information was relayed to the appropriate health care providers. Regular weekly sessions were held in community pharmacies, and continuity of care was enhanced through explicit links between pharmacists and family physicians.

In a number of mid-sized towns in Canada, the authors trained volunteers to measure blood pressure accurately and assess other cardiovascular risk. These volunteers then held education sessions for a period of 10 weeks in the pharmacies where they were stationed. As clients 65 or older walked in, the volunteer asked if they would be willing to participate in the program for 10 weeks, and if agreeable, their blood pressure was taken, they answered questions about other vascular risk factors they may have, and they attended the education sessions. By prior agreement, if the individual's blood pressure was too high, they were either sent to their family physician or to the emergency room.

The results the authors monitored included hospital admissions for heart attacks and stroke and congestive heart failure in the year before this program started, and compared the results with the data from the year after CHAP was implemented.

They concluded that CHAP was associated, within one year, with a 9% relative reduction in hospital admissions due to strokes and cardiovascular diseases, simply by educating individuals about what the risk factors are, what each individual can do about it, and maintaining the program for 10 weeks. That is a lot of citizens whose health improved with a small investment of time, and they remained working productively and available to their families.

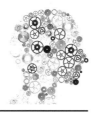

RULE 4

Eat Right, Weigh Light, and Stay Bright!

Food is essential for life . . . but only in moderation. Too much of it will have grave consequences on your physical and mental health, as this chapter will outline. Even the ancients recognized that overeating can be harmful. There was a saying among them that "we should start eating only when we are hungry, and we should stop eating before we are full." In our modern Western society, not only is there emphasis on eating a lot, but the food we eat often packs many calories.

Obesity has many negative effects on our health, not the least of which is that it is a driver of dementia, so the growing epidemic of obesity in most of the world is particularly worrisome. This chapter describes the dimensions of the problem and the causes of obesity in the world. It also provides tried and true advice on how we can individually overcome this problem.

I want to state categorically that I do not make moral judgements about obese individuals. My only desire is to explain the condition so that they are aware of the reasons for and conse-quences of obesity. I think of obesity as a medical problem that negatively affects health in general and the brain in particular, and I want to be firmly supportive of any obese person who is concerned about their condition and wants to do something about it.

How Can I Assess If I Am Overweight or Obese?

Deciding whether you need to do something about your weight starts by figuring out how overweight you are—or if your weight falls into a healthy range. To do this, you need some information. One popular tool is the body mass index (BMI), which is a simple calculation using a person's height and weight. You start by measuring your height. As we age, we shrink, so you can't rely on how tall you used to be. We need to measure how tall we are once a year or so past the age of 60 to get an accurate reading of our height. The next step is to weigh yourself on a scale.

With those two measurements, you can calculate your BMI:

- The formula is BMI = kg/m^2 where kg is a person's weight in kilograms and m^2 is their height in metres multiplied by itself. If you know your height only in inches and your weight in pounds, no problem. Calculate your BMI using the following formula:

$$\frac{\text{Weight (lbs) x 703}}{\text{Height (inches) x Height (inches)}} = \text{BMI in kg/m}^2$$

- A BMI of 25.0 or more is overweight, and obesity is defined as a BMI of 30 or more; the healthy range is 18.5 to 24.9. BMI applies to adults over the age of 18. (See more at www.diabetes.ca/diabetes-and-you/healthy-living-resources/weight-management/body-mass-index-bmi-calculator#sthash.xU3SQUR5.dpuf.)

While BMI is a better index than weight alone to determine if you are overweight, it is not perfect because it does not take the shape of our bodies into account. If you are muscular instead of obese, or if the fat is concentrated around the middle, BMI is insensitive to these important variations. For this reason, an additional new way to assess our health in relation to our weight is to measure waist circumference, as there is a direct correlation between waist circumference and the tendency to have diabetes, elevated cholesterol, and hardening of the arteries, all of which affect brain health.[1] Waist circumference may be a more accurate measure of our health status: waistlines in U.S. adults expanded by 1 inch from 2000 to 2012 but their BMI did not change much.[2] Simply measure your waist circumference just above the top of the hip bones, and use that value to assess obesity: it should be 50% or less of your height. So if you are a male, to help stay healthy you want to have a BMI of less than 25 kg/m^2 and a waist circumference of less than 102 cm (40 inches). For best overall health for women, the waist circumference should be less than 88 cm (35 inches). Depending on how much higher your two measurements are, your overall health will be at increased risk, at high risk, or at very high risk.

It is important to remember that these figures apply to Caucasian men and women. For example, whereas a Caucasian male can have a waist circumference of up to 101.6 cm (40 inches) before being considered at high risk for developing health problems, for a South Asian, Chinese or South American male, the cut-off is 88 cm (35 inches).

The Consequences of Obesity

Obesity in preschool children can have many unfortunate long-term consequences. It can lead to chronic health problems as well as social challenges and poor academic performance.[3] Obesity reprograms the brain. Brain regions that signal "You are now full so please stop eating" are not as active in the brains of obese individuals as they are in those of non-obese people, while regions that signal "Hey I deserve a food reward" are more easily activated. Also, the diet consumed during the adolescent years has a major determining effect on subsequent food tastes and may explain the difficulty in maintaining weight-loss programs when obesity develops later.[4] A high-fat diet in the early years turns down the reward regions of the brain so that more high-calorie food is needed to provide the same degree of pleasure. As well, obesity alters the gustatory perception of food so that a preference for fatty foods is acquired.[5] This may explain why providers of high-calorie foods claim they are simply providing what their customers want.

Obesity rewires your brain to perpetuate the condition, and food companies think of obese children as their guarantee of a future revenue stream. That is why it takes enormous willpower to lose weight. Losing weight is one of the hardest things to do, despite hype that it can be easy. So perhaps it would help to describe the negative effect of obesity on our health as a way of encouraging us to get on with battling it.

Let me start by stating categorically that there is no such thing as "healthy obesity." Many experts now consider obesity to be a disease. Studies have shown that obese individuals are eight times more likely to develop health problems over time than normal-weight individuals. They are more likely to develop type 2 diabetes, high blood pressure, and abnormalities in cholesterol. Nor is the excess fat that an obese person carries, particularly around the abdomen, an inert substance. This visceral fat is a metabolically active extra "organ" that secretes nasty pro-inflammatory chemicals into the bloodstream. Thus one harmful consequence of obesity is that it weakens the immune system, which has a detrimental effect on our blood vessels and weakens their ability to dilate or constrict in response to the metabolic needs of the brain.[6] One study found that when one particular pro-inflammatory compound (interleukin-6) was elevated on two occasions over a period of five years, it halved the individual's chances of aging well, with a significant increase in the incidence of heart disease, diabetes, and even some cancers.[7] There is also a proven strong relationship between excessive BMI and an elevation in blood pressure,[8] and the complications of obesity have now been confirmed to include strokes, both the overt and covert varieties.

Going to the core of what this book is about, there is also a positive correlation between an elevated BMI and dementia, shown in many studies: the Honolulu-Asia Aging Study[9] and Xu and colleagues in the journal *Neurology*[10] are just two of these studies. A 2013 study found that obese individuals had more trouble with executive functions,[11] and a few years earlier, another study showed that those carrying extra abdominal fat tended to have lower brain volume.[12] Therefore, either directly or through its impact on blood pressure and increased stroke incidence, excessive weight will eventually contribute to cognitive impairment and dementia.

As mentioned, one of the more serious complications of obesity is type 2 diabetes. This condition is becoming more prevalent, like obesity itself, in every country in the world. In Canada more than 3 million individuals are already affected by this condition, and children are developing type 2 diabetes at an increasing rate. The complications of diabetes are long term: untreated diabetes accelerates arterial disease and creates a toxic environment for our brains. This is in addition to its negative consequences on the blood supply to our kidneys, often requiring chronic dialysis; on our limbs, requiring in extreme cases amputations to avoid gangrene; and on our reproductive systems, leading to sexual dysfunction. Diabetes that is not controlled will negatively affect thinking, memory, and other aspects of cognition, and even before any of its complications such as strokes are evident, mental decline is often noticeable, confirming the toxicity of diabetes to the brain. This association between diabetes and dementia was confirmed in a study of 1 million people followed in Taiwan for 11 years.[13] It showed that diabetic patients experienced a higher incidence of dementia than non-diabetic patients. Some dietary changes, such as the Mediterranean diet, that help improve cognitive difficulties work only if the individual does not already suffer from diabetes, which implies that the risk to our minds imposed by diabetes is so great that dietary manipulations alone are unable to overcome the risk. As well, those with diabetes wanting to prevent strokes will need to follow more stringent guidelines for the control of blood pressure and cholesterol levels. This extra level of care recognizes the fact that diabetes itself is potentially so harmful that other risk factors must be further reduced as a consequence.

The mechanisms that link fatty and sugar-rich diets to memory difficulty were recently described in an article that reviewed all the relevant literature in this area.[14] It confirmed a report from Australia showing that animals fed fatty and sweet foods showed inflammation in the brain areas associated with memory functions, making them less able to function.

A number of other reports showed that the fine structure of blood vessels feeding the memory sites in the brain deteriorates in a high-glucose environment.[15]

Perhaps the best proof for the impact of obesity on our cognitive abilities is, perversely, obtained from individuals who undergo bariatric surgery, surgery that aims at reducing the size of the stomach. More than 100 patients who underwent this surgery were studied for their cognitive function.[16] Prior to the surgical intervention, 24% of these patients exhibited impaired learning performance and 23% had difficulty with recognition memory. Twelve weeks post-surgery, the performance of these individuals on these tests normalized. This is evidence that obesity has a significant negative impact on our ability to remember, think, and make decisions and good judgements, but the good news is that its impact is potentially reversible if we slim down before too much damage is sustained by the memory pathways in our brain.

The Good, Bad, and Deadly in Our Diet

The Good

When Rick Gallop was the CEO of the Heart and Stroke Foundation of Ontario, he was concerned about the issue of obesity worldwide. During his tenure, studies confirmed the negative impact of obesity on vascular health, so he decided to do something about it. He expanded the concept of the glycemic index and wrote a book titled *The G.I. Diet*. He assigned traffic-light colours to different foods depending on their glycemic index number. Items with a high glycemic index were red, meaning the item has a high sugar content that the body rapidly absorbs so you feel hungry quickly after you consume it. Green indicated items with a low glycemic index—you could eat them without being concerned about their weight effect. Items in the orange column were those you could consume with moderation. The goal of the book was to help individuals lose weight without feeling too hungry and lower the risk of heart disease, stroke, and diabetes. He also recommended portion control by specifying that half our dinner plate should be filled with greens or vegetables; a quarter only with a meat, preferably fish or chicken; and the last quarter with a carbohydrate like potatoes (not fries) or rice.

There are other good suggestions for diet that are now proven to be healthy. The DASH diet (Dietary Approaches to Stop Hypertension) was developed by the National Institutes of Health in the United States with the aim of lowering blood pressure without medication.[17] The diet has the added benefit of reducing cholesterol in the blood. It is rich in fruits, vegetables, and low-fat or non-fat dairy; emphasizes a reduction in refined grains in favour of whole grains; and promotes lean meats, fish, and poultry. Most importantly, the diet limits the amount of salt consumed. Following the DASH diet results in improvement in executive function, memory, and learning as well as speed of thinking. When combined with a weight management program and aerobic exercise, the DASH diet improves cognitive function in those who suffer from high blood pressure.[18]

The Mediterranean diet has also had recent scientific confirmation of its ability to decrease the likelihood of dementia.[19] Perhaps related to this is the proven benefit of the Mediterranean diet in reducing the likelihood of diabetes by as much as 40%.[20] Those who adhere to this diet can also expect to live longer,[21] and even when people who follow this diet pay no attention to calories, they still have a lower incidence of obesity and diabetes.[22] On the other end of the spectrum, individuals with normal cognition who do not adhere to the Mediterranean diet show a thinner ribbon of grey matter in their brains, perhaps foreshadowing trouble to come.[23]

The essential features of the Mediterranean diet are as follows:

- An abundance of fruits, vegetables, legumes, nuts

- Whole grain cereals and whole grain breads

- Extra virgin olive oil as the primary source of fat

- Low intake of saturated fat and no trans fats

- Low amounts of dairy products

- Fish, poultry, and eggs a few times a week

- Red meat only a few times a month

- A moderate amount of wine with meals

As you see, in addition to recommending a lot of vegetables, fruits, nuts, and fish, the diet uses olive oil for cooking, which has the highest percentage (77%) of monounsaturated fat of all the oils, including butter and margarine. The expected impact of following this eating plan would be to reduce vascular disease such as hypertension, and there is now evidence that eating this way on a regular basis reduces the likelihood of developing memory and cognitive difficulties.[24]

The Mediterranean diet also seems to confer long life by decreasing the likelihood of cancer and heart disease. A study conducted recently in Boston included a review of the health records of 120,000 patients and showed that those who consumed nuts of any variety (pistachios, peanuts, almonds) were 20% less likely to die during the study, 11% less likely to get cancer, 29% less likely to get heart disease, and more likely to be slim—all from eating a handful of nuts per day.[25] The concern that nuts contain high calories and will make you fat was dealt a blow by this study, probably because snacking on nuts increases your sense of being full, leading to lower consumption of other potentially nastier calories in chips or candy. In fact, a review of relevant studies in this field found that most often, adults who eat nuts weigh less than nut avoiders.[26] Additionally, nuts contain healthy unsaturated fats and several other healthy non-fat constituents. If you're still concerned about the high caloric content of nuts, go for nuts in the shell so you cannot just grab a handful and pop them in your mouth.

The Bad

We all lead hectic lives, and often due to lack of time and as a reward for a hard day's work, we drive to a fast food joint and grab some food to take home. You may remember the story of Mr. T., related earlier. Let's look at that for a minute. If Mr. T. stopped at a hamburger joint on his way home and bought a sandwich like a Big Mac, he'd be purchasing 550 calories; if he got a quarter-pounder with cheese, that's 520. If he brought home four pieces of fried chicken, he'd have more than 2,000 calories in the box. In addition to the calories, fast food meals are likely high in saturated fats, salt, and sugar, especially if the meal is accompanied by a soft drink. As well, if Mr. T. was determined not to do any shopping, he and his family were likely not eating many fruits and vegetables as snacks.

A recent report from the Center for Science in the Public Interest, a Washington-based advocacy group, reviewed the changes in the American diet from 1970 to 2010.[27] It revealed that Americans still consumed more beef and pork than chicken and fish, with the average person in 2010 consuming annually 20 pounds more in total fat than he or she did in 1970. Interestingly, the comment was made that Americans think that if a food is considered healthier, you can eat a lot of it! We may all be guilty of this kind of thinking, but it is important to remember that olive oil, for instance, admittedly a much healthier alternative than butter or lard because it has much more unsaturated fat, still packs the same number of calories as those alternatives for the same weight! That's why it is important to pick good fats for our diet.

And the Deadly...

Food bought in fast food outlets seems to have become increasingly packed with more and more calories. A meal offered recently at the Canadian National Exhibition in Toronto was a hybrid between a doughnut and a croissant, called a Cronut Burger. When all the sides and drinks that went with the meal were added in, it clocked in at 7,500 calories! That is the equivalent of more than three days' worth of calories in one meal. In some of the southern states, a new kind of dessert is chocolate-covered bacon! These are just two examples of excess in the prepared foods we can buy. When the owners of the restaurant offering the Cronut Burger were asked about this meal, they said they were simply offering what people were asking for. There is an unfortunate emphasis on "bigness" among some young people, and the market is responding.

In North America, the volume of food consumed has gone up significantly over time, and the industrial methods of food production have made it possible to buy large quantities of processed food at reasonable prices. We tend to "supersize" everything. We offer double and triple patties in hamburgers, and pasta bowls are advertised as "never ending." Even fresh fruit and vegetables suffer—modern peaches and strawberries may be large, but they are also less tasty.

Too Much Fat

The Cronut Burger was made up of two ground-bacon patties, a slice of peameal bacon, crispy bacon strips, and cheddar. This came accompanied by a side of bacon-cheese fries and a peanut butter and bacon milkshake. Every single component in the meal was laden with saturated fats, the most harmful variety. There are basically three kinds of fats: saturated, mono-unsaturated, and polyunsaturated:

1. The saturated fats come mostly from animal fats but are also found in oils from tropical foods such as coconut. No more than 6% of your total caloric intake should come from these fats.

2. Olive oil is the most common monounsaturated fat, but others in this category include canola and sunflower as well as oils derived from or contained in nuts. Provided we use them in moderation, monounsaturated oils will suppress the bad cholesterol in our blood. This is thought to partly explain why the Mediterranean diet reduces cardiovascular risk.

3. Polyunsaturated fats are where all the omega varieties reside. Healthy polyunsaturated oils would have equal omega-6 and omega-3 components. Unfortunately, we eat a lot more omega-6 oils, which come from corn, and fewer omega-3 oils, which come from fish. The omega-6 oils have increasingly found their way into our diet, particularly in processed foods, because changes in government subsidies in the United States made corn oil plentiful and cheap. Other sources of omega-6 oils are cottonseed, which is used mainly in the Middle East, and soybean. Recent research has shown that increasing omega-3 fatty acid

intake has a positive effect on cognition, particularly in people suffering from mild cognitive impairment.[28]

The unhealthy fat that we should completely avoid is trans unsaturated fats (trans fats). Compared to saturated fats, trans fats pose far greater health risks. As mentioned before, saturated fats are mostly animal fats, found in foods such as egg yolk, salmon, and red meat. Trans fats are found in processed foods, such as margarine. These fats are primarily industrially made and their main purpose is to help increase the shelf life of these products. A recent review of 41 studies examined the association between saturated or trans fats intake and health outcomes. While it was found that consuming saturated fats was not connected to heart disease, stroke, or diabetes, the consumption of trans fats was associated with a 34% increase in all-cause mortality, a 28% increased risk of heart disease mortality, and a 21% increase in risk of heart disease![29] Trans fats are definitely not good for you!

Luckily, it is easy to limit consumption of trans fats with a little preparation and insight into what you are eating. The nutritional facts label on the back of consumer foods is an effective tool for determining what is in your food. The amount of trans fat in a product is listed under this label. Keep a lookout for "partially hydrogenated oils" in the ingredients as well. Even if the product says trans fat–free, if it contains partially hydrogenated oils, it is a source of trans fat. Some foods to avoid are packaged snack foods and ready-made baked goods, such as cookies or pastries, frozen meals and entrées, cake mixes, and microwave popcorn.

A growing trend in North America is to "fatten" even the healthiest foods. Fish that is grilled, baked, or broiled is a very healthy food item, and while I enjoy the occasional fish and chips, eating battered fish increases the caloric content significantly and negates the benefits of eating the healthier food.

I recommend using olive oil in cooking and on salads as dressing. Increase fish intake without frying it because of its high omega-3 content. Walnuts and other nuts, which are recommended additions to your diet, are also high in omega-3 oils.

Too Much Salt

On average, we consume much more salt than the recommended level. More than 70% of the salt we consume comes from purchased processed food, restaurant food, and packaged consumable items. And extra salt brings more trouble: a recent study showed that in a nationally representative sample of U.S. children, the average sodium intake was 3056 mg per day (equivalent to 7.8 g of salt per day), and the more salt was consumed the more sugar-sweetened beverages were drunk, compounding the problem of obesity.[30] Remember that the Canadian Stroke Network and other organizations recommend limiting our salt intake to 1500 mg of sodium per day from all food sources.

Too Much Sugar

Since the 1970s, the average percentage of daily calories taken in from sugary drinks in North America has more than doubled. Despite this, the sugar derived from drinks represents only a third of all the sugar that a North American consumes—the rest of it comes from sugar in processed foods like breads, jams, ice cream and cakes, and canned food items such as salad dressings, tomato sauce, and cereals.[31]

Not that this absolves soft drinks! A 2013 report showed that drinking one or more cans of sugary drinks a day is associated with an increase in the risk of diabetes in later life, confirming that consuming sugary drinks is associated with obesity.[32] A more recent study reported that 1% of Japanese deaths but 30% of Mexican deaths under the age of 45 could be attributed to sugary drinks. The study also found that 25,000 deaths annually may be attributable to sweetened drinks in the United States.[33]

The Drivers of the Obesity Epidemic

The unfortunate physiological reality, as mentioned earlier, is that eating meals laden with fat and packed with calories modifies the appetite and pleasure centres in our brains so that it is more difficult to shed the excess weight. In fact, 7% of women and 3% of men admit that they are addicted to food, meaning they eat to the point of feeling physically ill.[34] This is likely the driver behind the comment made by the Cronut Burger creators: they were simply offering the public what it was asking for.

The greatest growth in obesity occurred in rich countries or countries where the standard of living recently improved. For this reason, some have suggested that improved incomes allow individuals to choose, and advertising directs them towards, more processed foods they can easily afford. The higher standards of living also move people to city centres, accelerating urbanization and leading to a more sedentary lifestyle. Perhaps the best evidence for the association of improved economic status with obesity is what is going on in Qatar. Qatar, now the world's fattest country, is the world's wealthiest nation.[35]

Some of us have responded to the challenge of maintaining a healthy weight by going for diet drinks that contain sweeteners. It is true that these contain fewer calories, but when you drink diet pop, two things happen:

1. You may feel "diet-virtuous" and give yourself permission to consume calories later, sometimes many more than you would have if you had avoided the diet drink in the first place. This phenomenon actually has a name. It is called cognitive distortion, meaning we can convince ourselves that splurging is okay because our drinks were low calorie.

2. You will likely feel hungry sooner. Aspartame, the ingredient in most diet drinks, is excessively sweet, but it has no calories, so the brain seeks to compensate by generating a rebound feeling of hunger sooner.

Finally, for many of us in society, food has come to mean comfort. For some, food is not just physically satisfying but emotionally fulfilling. It makes up for being alone, for feeling lonely, for feeling emotionally bereft. A very full stomach comforts a lonely heart. I know of no statistics to back up this statement, but I believe the confirmed rise in the sense of loneliness, which we will talk about later, fuels the growth in our girth. It is important to be aware of this link if we are to understand the drivers of the epidemic of obesity in society.

Despite all these challenges, when we decide to shed the excess pounds, it takes single-minded determination to succeed...but success is possible.

Attitudes and Behaviours That Favour Weight Reduction and Control

If it were easy to slim down and maintain a healthy body weight, many more of us would be slim. Nonetheless, it is very much worth a try. Even modest weight loss, say losing just 5% of body weight, has many positive health benefits.

There is also good news about the nasty visceral or abdominal fat: it is fat that is particularly vulnerable to melting away in response to exercise.[36]

Unfortunately, in my clinical experience, there is no easy way to lose weight. To wilfully deprive yourself of food you like or are used to involves a difficult choice between pleasure now and health later. It usually takes an unhappy event or incident to muster the willpower to launch a weight-loss program and maintain it. For some, it is a dress that does not fit anymore, perhaps a snide comment made intentionally or otherwise about one's looks, or the start of one of the many consequences of obesity, such as a knee that now makes walking painful or an elevated blood sugar that the doctor tells you presages diabetes. Whatever the trigger, if you have decided to shed the extra pounds, congratulations on preferring health to disease, and read on!

Once you've made up your mind, it is important to remember that there is no sure method guaranteed to result in weight loss. However, there seem to be three successful ways to lose weight:

1. A sudden thorough break with past eating habits. Men often follow this path to weight loss. Suddenly, old eating habits and diets are abandoned, and one of the diets recommended earlier is adopted and followed for life.

2. The slow route, which in my experience is frequently followed by women who are determined to lose weight. They may join Weight Watchers or follow their online version, or moderate their current eating habits by cutting out a few egregious items. Social support is essential for success with this method.

3. Surgery to band the stomach (bariatric surgery). This is the brutal route to weight loss, leading to shrinking the size of the stomach and making it difficult (but not impossible) to consume large quantities of food.

In fact, how you get to the point of being absolutely determined to succeed in your weight-loss goal does not really matter. Professional help is extremely useful, and in some situations essential.

The Steps to Successful Weight Loss

After reviewing many studies, I have concluded that weight-loss success is more likely if the following steps are taken:

1. The weight-loss program is started only when you have absolute and deep determination to protect your health and future cognitive functions. Start only when you're determined to succeed and have the strong conviction that *only* diet modification can achieve weight loss. Be sure to start by assessing and understanding what in your diet and lifestyle combined have brought you to where you are.

2. Make sure you have social support while pursuing the difficult goal of shedding pounds. A study has shown that in-person support and even support delivered remotely without face-to-face contact has resulted in obese patients achieving and sustaining significantly more weight loss than control subjects who got no support.[37] Support may also be available from the community. Regardless, you need someone or a number of individuals who will take interest and provide support, follow-up, and feedback.

3. When you are good and ready, do not set unrealistic goals. Your challenge is to modify your behaviour more than count calories. Do not start by defining the weight-loss goal or target weight, as these mental set-points are a recipe for disappointment and lead people to give up on their weight-loss program. Instead, adopt a proven diet such as the glycemic index or the Mediterranean diet, and remember that portion control is key: it doesn't matter how healthy your diet is, if you eat too much, you will put on weight. The good news is that the rate at which you lose weight will not affect whether later you will regain some of it, so go for it.

4. Do not skip meals. Eat breakfast, ideally fruits. During the day, consume healthy snacks. Those who have lost weight successfully have reported that keeping their tummies happy frequently led them to eat smaller main meals. And if you have an absolute favourite food item, regardless of its caloric content, continue to eat small amounts of it so you don't feel you have been totally deprived of something you enjoy.

5. Resolve to substitute nutritious food for unhealthy varieties. I stated that the brains of obese individuals have a preference for fatty foods, but the brain can be retrained to prefer healthy foods.[38] With the Mediterranean diet you will increase the proportion of fruits, vegetables, and seafood you consume. I suggest you eat fish or other seafood three times a week, and decrease the amount of red meat to once a week, then eat chicken one to two days a week. In the remaining day or two in the week, eat dishes that include chickpeas, beans, or lentils—all of which have been proven in the

context of the Mediterranean diet to have great health benefits.

6. When you eat chicken or fish, take the skin off, and remember that meat that is "marbled" means you will consume extra fat. Strip as much fat off your smaller piece of meat as you can before you cook it. Do not fry anything, and do not eat anything that is breaded then cooked in fat. Avoid any meat that is "flavoured" or marinated. These are excuses for adding salt to the meat, which is then not only unhealthy, but costs more as you are paying for the water the extra salt holds on to.

7. Make sure your *daily* intake of fruit includes at least five different fruits. Ideally, colourful fruits are part of your choice because they have been shown to lower blood pressure and have a number of other health benefits, but any fruit will do. I grant you that it is more expensive to buy fresh fruits and vegetables than to buy canned ones, but I want you to think of the increased cost as an investment in your brain's future health.

8. Snack carefully. If you find some foods impossible to resist snacking on (like ice cream or cake), resolve not to buy them so you are not tempted by them. Make fruit your preferred snack. Snacking on crisp vegetables such as celery sticks or carrots can be refreshing, and they have a low glycemic index. But be careful with dressings and sauces: some of them pack a wallop of calories, so make sure you are not neutralizing the benefits of eating vegetables by adding too many calories in dressings and sauces.

9. Another excellent snack is a few nuts of your choice. Make sure they are unsalted and ideally in the shell. Finally, don't

snack on anything from a shiny bag! All your food should be as close to what nature created as possible, meaning you should avoid processed foods.

10. Avoid "all you can eat" buffets. It is well-proven that under these circumstances the glutton in us is awakened and becomes an insatiable beast. Also, avoid shopping on an empty stomach. Those who do purchase items with higher calorie content than those who eat a small snack prior to shopping.[39]

11. Consuming some alcohol before or during a meal encourages increased calorie consumption from food.[40] Alcohol consumption is a double-edged sword: a drink a day is in fact helpful in reducing some vascular risk factors because it dilates and relaxes blood vessels, but more alcohol than that is not only a significant cause of weight gain but has a direct negative impact on cognition.

12. Don't buy and eat food while sitting in your car at a drive-through window. It is a wasted opportunity to neutralize some of the calories. Park a distance away, walk to the joint at a fast clip, and then order your food. That will at least get you up to burn some calories, but it is best to avoid calorie-laden fast foods.

13. Take the salt shaker off the table! Most vegetables have salt in them naturally, and if you eat them fresh, that is all you need. Beware, though: if you currently consume a lot of salt and you suddenly cut back, food will taste flat. But after about three weeks, if someone puts back the salt you used to use, you will find the food incredibly salty. Our taste buds require some time to adjust up or down to the amount of salt we consume. So go for it: take the

salt shaker off the table, don't sprinkle salt on your food, and just be patient for a while.

It's Not Only What We Eat—How We Eat Also Matters

We do not eat just to fill the space in our belly called the stomach. We also eat to satisfy our brain. Eating is hardwired in our brains as the reward for productive work. It is therefore important to take the time to taste and enjoy the food. Yes, sometimes we have only a few minutes for our lunch and grab some sustenance, but even in that setting it is crucial to savour and enjoy our food. It is not enough for the food to fill our stomach; it has to satisfy our soul!

At the beginning of 2014, various specialists were asked "What is the one thing people can do to be healthier this year?" I like what Dr. Arya Sharma had to say: "If you spend less than 60 minutes a day eating, you are eating too fast. It takes at least 20 minutes for your gut to tell your brain that you've eaten. Paying attention to what you are eating, chewing and savouring each bite, eating without distractions such as driving or phone calls or texting, all go a long way to reduce overeating."

I have seen how some of us go against this crucial rule. Some individuals will cut a morsel of food, and no sooner have they put it in their mouth than their utensil is busy preparing the next bite. While they are doing that, they do not taste what is in their mouth, and their mind is not registering the fact that they are eating. They are fully focused on the next morsel. That is a recipe for overeating. I strongly recommend that you eat mindfully: after you put a bite of food in your mouth, put down the utensil, focus your mind on tasting what you are chewing and enjoying, then pick up the utensil to take the next morsel only after you have swallowed what is in your mouth. You will find that you don't eat as much, feel full sooner, and enjoy your food more. A recent study confirmed that those who eat slower consume fewer calories.[41] Someone has even invented a fork called HapiFork that turns red and vibrates if you pause it less than 10 seconds between two trips to your mouth!

Another habit that is very detrimental to our health is "double-tasking" while we are eating. Some of us eat our breakfast absentmindedly while reading the morning headlines or checking emails that came in overnight. Others have supper while watching TV or using the computer. Eating while your brain is busy with some other activity goes against the essential rule of mindful eating. It will deprive your mind of the sense of satisfaction that comes from consuming food. Consequently, your stomach is full but your mind is hungry, and you will be looking to satisfy your mental need for food.

Eating Excessively Cannot Be Neutralized by Exercise

Is there anything wrong with eating more than you need if you can "burn" the excess calories through exercise? No, there is nothing wrong with that in theory, but in practice, it just doesn't work. A friend of mine used to visit his favourite French bakery on weekends for a latte and an almond croissant. He was dismayed to learn that the calories in that single meal nullified almost all his caloric expenditure through exercise during the week.

Here are some of the activities the consumer of that Cronut burger would have to do in order to "burn" 7,500 calories:

▸ Running at 7 miles an hour for 8 hours

- ▸ Cycling leisurely for 23 hours

- ▸ Vigorously rowing for 10.7 hours

To get full details on how many calories are burned by specific activities, go to nutristrategy.com/caloriesburned.htm.

For most of us there just isn't time or will to make that kind of heroic commitment to exercise. Exercise simply does not burn off as many calories as we desperately want to believe it does. The best way to keep the pounds off is not to put them on in the first place, but I do wish you success in getting to or maintaining a healthy weight.

How Big Is the Problem of Obesity?

All of us, regardless of where we live in the world, have been getting fatter. Consequently, in the United States, almost 70% of men and women are overweight (BMI of 25 kg/m² or more) and half of the population satisfies the criteria for obesity (BMI of 30 kg/m² or more). In 2009, 25% of Canadian men and 23% of Canadian women satisfied the criteria for obesity. In the developing world, over the past 30 years, the number of obese and overweight individuals has multiplied 4-fold and now rests at 1 billion individuals. These are distressing figures.

As if this was not bad enough, the worse news is what is going on with our youth. Statistics in Canada show that in the 10 years from 1994 to 2005 there was a 19% increase in obesity in the 12 to 34 age group, and a 20% increase in obesity in the 35 to 39 age group. Boys aged 12 to 34 increased their rate of obesity in those 10 years by 40%.

Children have a tendency to begin putting on weight around the age of six, but if they overeat at earlier times, they will show excessive weight gain at even younger ages. More importantly, children who put on weight excessively or do so at earlier ages have a much higher chance of becoming obese adults, and they are more likely to also suffer from high blood pressure and high levels of fat in their bloodstreams.

Figure 8 shows a diagram I developed that summarizes the consequences of obesity and the factors that lead to its development.

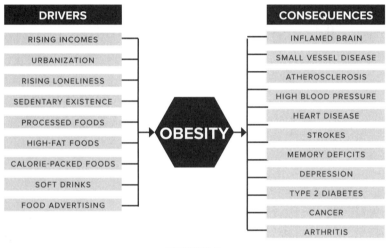

FIGURE 8

Drivers and health consequences of obesity

Many factors listed on the left contribute to obesity. Unfortunately, those of us who are overweight may suffer a number of health consequences, shown on the right.

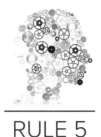

RULE 5

Move Your Hind ... to Save Your Mind

There is now strong evidence that being physically active prevents your brain from melting away! In this chapter, you will learn how much physical activity you need and which exercises are more likely to maintain brain vitality. The chapter will also provide suggestions on how an active life can become part of your daily routine and decrease or even replace the need for formal exercising. I will also touch on the potential harmful effects of excessive and sudden physical activity.

What Is the Problem We Are Trying to Solve?

A confluence of factors has led us to move our bodies far less than we need and exercise our minds less than we require. These factors are sometimes referred to as "civilization." Many of us have less than adequate sleep, get up and drive to work (sitting), have an office where we work (sitting), have a lunch break (sitting), drive back home (sitting), and after we sit at supper, we sit down and work at our desk, or sit down on a comfortable chair and watch TV, read the paper, or catch up on emails and texting. It is estimated that 48% of adult Canadians are inactive, and Americans older than 65 watch on average 4 hours and 40 minutes of TV a day. Only 10% of them walked an hour a day, the remainder walking less than that. A survey performed in the United Kingdom in 2013 showed that a quarter of its citizens walked no more than one hour in an entire week, and another 40% walked less than two hours per week.[1] A more recent survey of 2,000 office workers in the United Kingdom showed that 45% of women and 37% of men spent less than 30 minutes a day on their feet at work.[2]

Not only do modern life's demands reduce the opportunities for walking and moving, but avoiding physical activity has become ingrained in our psyche and our behaviour. Isn't the photograph in figure 9 a sad commentary on how absurdly attached we have become to avoiding physical activity, even when we are seeking it?

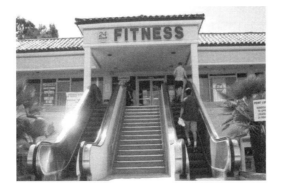

FIGURE 9

Why are these fitness fanatics using the escalator?

Probably the two individuals in the picture feel short on time, as we all do, and feel that taking the escalator will get them to their exercise activity sooner. They may also take the escalator because "it's there," but in doing so they are depriving their bodies of the opportunity to climb stairs. We are all rushed, want to be efficient, and search even subconsciously for a minute we can save here and there. I work in a busy hospital, and the crowd of people gathered in front of the elevators is usually quite large, often to go up just one or two floors. You have likely observed, and perhaps even are guilty of the same, that people will drive around and around in a shopping centre's parking lot looking for a parking spot close to the entrance rather than park where there is lots of room and walk vigorously to the entrance. And of course some of us drive to a window and order fast food that we eat sitting in our cars.

Why am I providing all these examples? Does all this sedentary existence have a negative impact on our mind? *Absolutely*. Table 2 in Rule 2 shows that the percentage of dementia attributed worldwide to physical inactivity is 12.7%, but in North America, 21% of the dementias may be attributed to physical inactivity and our sedentary existence. So I will try to give you pointers on how you could become a lot more active while respecting the fact that none of us have a lot of free time.

How Does Physical Activity Help My Mind, and How Much Activity Do I Need?

When you undertake physical activity, let's say aerobic activity such as climbing stairs or bicycling or walking fast, the muscles being worked demand more blood. In order for the arteries to supply this extra blood, they have to relax—open up as it were. During the physical exertion itself, your heart is pumping and your blood pressure will go up to supply blood to all your working organs, such as the muscles you are moving and your heart that is now beating faster. The payback occurs after the physical exertion: your resting blood pressure will go down because your blood vessels have relaxed, and your resting pulse will slow because your heart is in better shape.[3] I can usually tell if my patients lead a physically active lifestyle simply by feeling their pulse or listening to their heart rate with my stethoscope. The patient whose heart beats fast at rest is usually surprised when I say, "It sounds to me you may be a bit out of shape" and wants to know how I reached that conclusion. If we are sedentary, the arteries in our body are not relaxed, our hearts beat harder, and our blood pressure if sustained may stay elevated. You've read now that elevated blood pressure has major negative consequences to body and mind, and reduced blood pressure has significant benefits.

There are lots of additional health benefits to physical activity. Activated muscles use up glucose, so your blood glucose level stabilizes, reducing the likelihood of diabetes. As well, increasing physical activity so that it is part of your regular routine reduces the level of inflammation in the blood circulating in your body, which has enormous benefits to all your body organs, including your brain. Perhaps for these and other reasons, a recent article in the journal *Stroke* reports lower stroke rates in individuals who walk a lot.[4]

We still have a great deal to learn about how muscle activation connects with brain health, but there is no doubt that it does. Our muscles have conversations with our brain, particularly the memory centres, and when the muscles move, they influence the health of our brain in many positive ways. If our muscles move a lot, our brain is healthier, and if they don't, our brain, particularly the memory centres, tend to weaken and may even pack it in. Almost 20 years ago my laboratory showed that a stroke will be less damaging to the brain when the concentration of a compound called "brain-derived neurotrophic factor," or BDNF, is higher. It turns out that exercise leads to the activation of this same compound. This may provide one mechanism by which exercise improves cognitive function. When we are sedentary, the ability of our muscles to activate BDNF declines and the brain becomes more vulnerable to vascular injury and consequently cognitive difficulty. As well, when our muscles are not activated, they do not consume glucose, and diabetes becomes more likely.

Several studies have examined the relationship between exercise and BDNF. I will describe the results so you can appreciate what exercise can do.

Physical activity promotes the formation of BDNF. Dr. Joshua Yarrow and his colleagues looked at the effect of training on circulating levels of BDNF. Twenty healthy untrained college-age males underwent a five-week traditional or enhanced progressive resistance training. Following a bout of resistance exercise, BDNF levels in the blood increased by 32%. The authors concluded that resistance exercise induced a robust yet transient elevation of circulating BDNF, and progressive resistance training augmented this response.[5]

"So what?" you may ask. What is the role of BDNF? What does it do for us?

BDNF promotes brain repair and elevates our mood. Barbara Hempstead, a professor of medicine, and colleagues recently reviewed all the actions of BDNF.[6] We have already touched on BDNF's role in reducing stroke damage, a result that came out of my own research, but it does a lot more than that. BDNF promotes tissue regeneration and opposes the action of inflammation, thus protecting and keeping healthy the lining of the arterioles feeding our brain cells.

Importantly, not only does BDNF activity seem to protect our memory functions but it also affects mental health in many positive ways. BDNF seems to counteract anxiety and depression. A.A. Garza and his colleagues showed that both exercise and antidepressant medication enhance the production of BDNF in the hippocampus, the structure so essential for good memory function, and this was true regardless of age.[7] That discovery lends credibility to Simon Whitfield's story below and the work of Dr. Mike Evans, a professor and staff physician at St. Michael's Hospital in Toronto. Both connected exercise to mood elevation.

You can see how important it is to keep moving to increase the concentration of this compound in our system! Exercising and living an active lifestyle is the most effective mechanism for preserving youth, in both body and mind.

As I have mentioned, we thought until recently that the brain had a fixed number of cells we were born with and they could only decrease with age. We thought you could not replace what is lost and rebuild brain parts. We now know, however, that the brain has a store of stem cells that can be mobilized out of their storage sites and sent to where they are needed. And here is some news that has stunned the scientific community: exercise is an activator of this process of stem cell mobilization and migration.

Physical activity remodels the brain to the benefit of its owner. Studies also show that just as being active changes the brain beneficially, being inactive changes brain function in detrimental ways. The same study that showed the benefit of activity to the brain showed the negative impact of sedentary existence by reporting that a sedentary lifestyle weakens the part of the brain that controls blood pressure, leading to its elevation and making heart disease and strokes more likely.[8]

The benefit we derive from exercise and physical activity occurs at all ages. Children perform better in the classroom if they are physically active and the reverse is also true: children who are inactive grow to become middle-aged couch potatoes.[9] At the other end of the age spectrum, a 2012 study showed that physical activity in 70-year-olds reduced brain atrophy and increased the integrity of the white matter in their brains over the following three years.[10] From 1971 to 2009, 19,458 adults living in their communities were studied and their fitness level was correlated with their incidence of dementia. The study's authors concluded that higher midlife fitness levels are associated with a lower likelihood of developing dementia.[11] So being physically active stops your brain from shrinking, and brain shrinkage (atrophy) is associated with cognitive difficulty and is more prevalent in individuals with dementia. The benefit from exercise even crosses into our progeny: animal studies suggest that healthy parents pass on healthy DNA to their progeny.[12]

The benefit to our brains from exercise occurs quite soon after it is started. In a 2013 review of the medical literature, researchers reported on two studies that showed benefit to memory and executive function after only six months of exercise.[13] A more recent study measured blood flow to the brain and assessed thinking ability after only 12 weeks of riding a stationary bike or working out on a treadmill for only one hour three times a week. The researchers showed that thinking ability and blood flow to the brain improved within that 12-week period as did cardiovascular fitness.[14] Another recent study looked at brain scans of individuals aged 60 to 88 and confirmed improvements in total brain volume and the volume of the hippocampus following a 12-week exercise program. The physical activity consisted of 20 minutes a day of moderate exercise that resulted in some sweating but the subject could still carry on a conversation at the end of the exercise period—that is, they were only moderately out of breath.[15] Importantly, the benefit was not limited to normal individuals but was also seen in those who already had mild trouble with cognition.

The fact that exercise can actually improve cognitive function after difficulties have already started in this domain was confirmed recently by a research team that showed that 6 months of doing moderate-intensity walking for 60 minutes 3 times a week not only improved the cognitive functions of participants with MCI but also increased the size of the hippocampus on their scans.[16] When I started to keep up with the medical literature on the benefits of exercise, I would have expected that a few months of exercise was too short a period of time to see benefit to our brains, but there is now concordant data showing that the brain improves both structure and function within weeks of exercise onset. Exercise grows your brain! And while we recommend 30 minutes of vigorous activity, a more recent study showed that even 20 minutes a day of running will reduce the risk of dementia by 25%, and increasing that to 27 minutes a day reduced the risk by 40%.[17]

I recommend that you do 20 minutes of modest physical activity every day. Your brain will reward you by improving your memory ability and your other cognitive functions. And the hope is that you will make a commitment right now to moving your butt for 20 minutes every day, sufficiently vigorously to get slightly short of breath during the activity. I predict you will enjoy being active so much that you will want to make it part of who you are, not a drudgery you impose on yourself.

What Kind of Exercise Is Best for My Brain?

Many adults limit their exercise to running or aerobics. "In the last few years, it's been believed that aerobics has been the most beneficial type of exercise to fight off dementia," says Dr. Teresa Liu-Ambrose of the University of British Columbia. "We thought other types of exercise might also be helpful, but not a lot of people believed in it." So Dr Liu-Ambrose built the research evidence needed to win over the skeptics among researchers, policy makers, and seniors alike, about the merits of resistance training—lifting weights or using resistance bands, for instance—to maintain cognitive abilities.

In a 2010 study, Dr. Liu-Ambrose showed that 12 months of progressive resistance training once or twice a week had a greater impact on improving cognitive skills in older women than the same amount of balance and toning exercises.[18] Seniors are often hesitant to lift weights, however. "They're concerned about fractures or sprains. But, like everything else, with proper guidance, resistance training is perfectly safe," says Dr. Liu-Ambrose. "Resistance training is appealing because not every older adult has the mobility to take part in aerobics, or can walk for long periods. The more options we can give people for exercise, the better." Working with a communications company to promote the benefits of resistance training, Dr. Liu-Ambrose and her research team developed and tested two videos to promote the benefits of resistance training, as well as showing the exercises. The team has posted the videos on YouTube and distributes them to health care professionals and seniors' organizations. They have received requests from around the world for permission to duplicate the videos in other languages.

Different types of exercise seem to have beneficial effects on different brain functions. Weight lifting or resistance training improves associative memory—recalling the names of the guests when you are reminded that you were at a restaurant—while cardiovascular exercise such as walking fast or running appears to improve verbal memory. So physical activity in all its forms reduces our risk for heart disease and stroke and awakens mechanisms that lead to brain cell production, and once the cells get to the brain, physical activity contributes to the preservation of the cells and gives them longevity.

For the most robust brain health, you should incorporate both aerobic and resistance training, since each type targets different aspects of cognitive health, and there is evidence that doing both types of exercise in the same session increases muscle strength and the molecules that are generated from each variety of activity. Importantly, exercise does not just slow down the decline in brain function. It can actually improve brain function. It is never too late to increase your physical activity.

Exercise Benefits Mental Health as Well as Mind and Body

An active lifestyle benefits other aspects of your health too. We have already mentioned that physical activity is an effective way of lowering your blood sugar level and reducing your risk for diabetes. Physical activity also counters the weakening of the immune system that accompanies aging so you become more resistant to infections.[19] Resistance training increases lean body mass while cardiovascular training will improve the lipid profile in your blood, so combined, both forms of exercise will decrease your likelihood of suffering from diabetes, heart disease, and stroke.[20] In addition to all these potential benefits, an active lifestyle will dull appetite, reducing hunger pangs and helping with the battle against the bulge.

Most people also report getting a high from physical activity. Jogging for some is their "happy pill." High levels of sedentary behaviour are associated with lower self-esteem and less pro-social behaviour.[21] Simon Whitfield, an Olympic champion, reported recently that he retired from Olympic sport in 2013 when he realized he "just didn't have the fire or the desire to make the obsessive commitment to compete."[22] He then related the consequences of his sedentary existence: "I spent the summer with no real training plan and fell out of a routine. I slowly drifted away from the practice of a daily fitness and wellness routine. By the end of the summer my mood was dark, my sleep was patchy and my mental health, the happiness and joy we all need to thrive, was growing dim. I knew I had to do something." Simon then reports how he took up the sport of stand-up paddle boarding and found that physical activity is key to a calm mind.

Contrast this with a recent experience I had when I visited a home for aged people. Every elderly person had a wheelchair with their name written on it! I asked why and was told that in order to prevent them from falling and breaking a bone or a hip, each person upon arrival to the facility was asked not to walk but only use the wheelchair to get around. I thought what a shame: in the process of protecting their bones, we are breaking their minds!

"I Don't Have Time for Formal Exercise. Any Suggestions?"

It takes superhuman determination to say "I am going to use my lunch hour to sweat." Most people just don't have the time or the willpower to exert themselves at specified times. Joining a gym and visiting it regularly also takes determination that often abandons us when we are too tired after putting in a long day at work. Some people will start with good intentions but quickly lose interest. Others will exercise because they want to lose weight, but you can't stuff your face with high-calorie food and expect that exercise will help you control your weight. An exercise regimen is ideal, but you could also integrate more physical activity that you enjoy into your day. So how do we achieve a time-efficient more active lifestyle?

You don't have to exhaust yourself jogging or run the marathon to achieve the benefits of exercise. The 2008 Physical Activity Guidelines for Americans recommended a minimum of 150 minutes of moderate-intensity or 75 minutes of vigorous-intensity activity per week for substantial health benefits. So the minimum is a commitment to 20 minutes a day that will result in some sweating or breathlessness. Do you think you can afford 10 minutes twice a day to protect your mind from the ravages of old age? If you have been totally sedentary and decided to start being more active, start slowly, making small incremental increases in your activity levels. There have been many attempts at finessing the figures, but 10 minutes of modest activity twice a day is a safe and effective goal. Some fitness centres have reduced this to a 7-minute intense workout based on the notion that intensity matters as much as duration. A 2006 paper showed that a three-minute sequence on a stationary bike—30 seconds of punishing pedalling followed by a brief rest, repeated five or six times—led to the same vascular responses as 90 minutes of prolonged bike riding.[23] Another study found that three 10-minute brisk walks during the day reduced blood pressure just as much as a single 30-minute session and had better protective effects against later BP spikes.[24] Similarly, a study from China in 2013 compared arterial stiffness resulting from one 30-minute versus two 15-minute sessions on a stationary bike and showed that arterial relaxation lasted longer after the second short session. So, as you can see, regardless of what the scientists measure, being physically active for short durations—20 to 30 minutes a day in divided doses—improves the way our body uses energy and our mental and cognitive health.

When I advise patients about the benefits of walking, I occasionally get asked "I take my dog for a walk in the afternoon. Isn't that good enough?" My answer is this: When you take your dog for a walk, you are away from the fridge and off the couch. That is helpful. You are outside in changing scenery and hopefully smelling fresh air and enjoying nature. You may even run into a neighbour and socialize a bit. All of that is great, but scientists have shown that just walking leisurely for 30 minutes a day over a six-week period had no impact on blood pressure. If you want to maximize the benefit to your body and mind, try to get out of breath during the walk. That is the signal your body needs to really relax the blood vessels feeding your muscles, your lungs, and your heart; reduce your blood pressure; mobilize the stem cells in your brain; and reduce inflammation in your blood. That's great return from a small time investment.

What else can you do? You can make up your mind that you will maximize the daily opportunities to be physically active. Test a variety of physical activities to see which ones you enjoy more and integrate them into your day rather than setting aside time to do exercises. Here are some specific suggestions:

1. Avoid all escalators.

2. Take the stairs rather than elevators, in both directions, for anything less than five floors.

3. Park far away from the entrance of the shopping centre and walk fast, or better still, jog to the entrance.

4. Going for a cup of coffee or to your work cafeteria for lunch? How about jogging slowly, enough to get out of breath?

5. If you are an office worker, consider working out while you work, by using a treadmill desk or a bicycle desk. If you go that route, start with small commitments of time that increase gradually. British experts are now recommending that we stand at least two hours a day.

6. Whenever the phone rings, stand up then pick up the phone. Better yet, consider getting a desk that allows you to do your work standing up. If you spend two hours a day standing, you are doing what the experts now recommend!

7. When you are brushing your teeth, flossing, shaving your face, combing your hair, or taking a shower, get in the habit of doing some squats. Bend your knees as if you were going to sit down, and maintain that position until you get tired. Take a rest, and then repeat. This will strengthen your core muscles and those around your thighs and knees. And hey, it is free resistance training—it doesn't cost you any additional time.

8. Walk! Walking is a wonderful way to stay fit but, as mentioned, for maximum benefit it must be vigorous enough to get you slightly winded. You can do it any time, it costs nothing, and you can easily vary both the intensity and the duration of your walk to suit your schedule. Recent studies have shown that a walk in nature is a useful antidote to the negative thoughts that crawl into our minds occasionally, but if you live in a cold climate and you worry about slipping on ice and falling, walk inside the house or go mall walking.

9. Dr. Mike Evans, whom I mentioned earlier, gave his best annual advice to readers of the *Globe and Mail* in January 2014. He said, "There is a super expensive new drug coming out. It reduces heart disease by 60 percent, cancer by 27 percent, Alzheimer's by 50 percent and arthritis by 47 percent. It is now our best treatment for fatigue and low back pain. It cuts anxiety and depression by 48 percent, and people even lose weight on the stuff. Okay, it's not a pill. It's walking."

I am certain you can come up with additional ways to incorporate physical activity into your daily routine. To avoid getting bored, vary the activity you indulge in. Provided you enjoy doing it rather than feel it is an imposition, you can walk one day, bicycle another, and maybe jog a third, all the while incorporating some of the suggestions mentioned earlier into your daily routine. And here is the good news: regardless of whether you exercise regularly or not, if you keep physically active during the day, your risk for cardiovascular disease is almost 30% lower than your couch potato neighbour.

And finally, the answer to a question you may be too shy to ask: Is sexual activity considered cardiovascular exercise? You will be happy to know that the answer is yes. On average, men burn 100 calories during sex and women burn 70. For reference, that is equivalent to 11 minutes of jogging on a treadmill for men and almost 10 minutes for women.

Aren't you glad you asked?

How Soon Will These Things Become a Habit?

Any time you start something new—take a new route to get to work, decrease the salt in your diet, or take an active walk during lunch—it doesn't become a habit overnight. That's why so many good intentions evaporate after New Year's! It takes doing something new repeatedly for a period of five to six weeks before it becomes just "part of what you do." The reasons for this are not clear, but in the case of reduction in salt intake, you'll recall that our taste buds adjust downward, so after five or six weeks on the low-salt diet, going back to the amount of salt you used to use will make the food taste impossibly salty! So it is important to be persistent when you start a new exercise program, or you give up smoking, or you change to a healthy diet. You need to keep at it until your brain doesn't think of the activity as being new. That's when it becomes part of you.

While persistence is important, creating a habit requires that you are honest with yourself and set a realistic goal to start with. Aim low to start, congratulate yourself for meeting that goal, and then creep it up. If in your heart of hearts you think 20 minutes of physical activity per day is too long, start with 10. If you are not a morning person, don't plan to go to the gym at 5:30 a.m. Plan both the kind of activity and its timing for your maximum enjoyment if you are serious about making a habit of being more active.

Can I Combine Exercise with the DASH diet and Weight Management?

If you combine three factors that work synergistically to control blood pressure and keep it normal, your brain will thank you profusely and reward you with excellent memory! A group in the United States has studied this.[25] They took 124 individuals who suffered from high blood pressure and were sedentary and overweight and convinced them to take three corrective measures simultaneously: go on the DASH diet, combine it with exercise, and reduce their caloric intake. They then compared the cognitive powers of this group to a group that ate their usual diet and lived their usual lifestyle. Participants who combined the DASH diet with calorie restriction and weight management exhibited greater improvements in executive memory functions than those who stayed on their usual diet. A 2015 study from Finland went further and combined diet, exercise, cognitive training, and vascular risk monitoring and compared the results with those obtained with general non-specific health advice. Cognitive function actually improved in the group that received the multi-domain intervention.[26] So what are we all waiting for? Let's move our butts and improve our dietary habits to stay smart.

Do It, But Don't Overdo It

If you've been a couch potato but have decided you're going to do something about it to improve your brain health, fantastic— go for it. But don't go out and start running the marathon! I have seen patients who very rapidly pushed themselves physically beyond their habitual level of fitness or endurance and suffered strokes and heart attacks. One middle-aged sedentary man went biking with his teenage daughter. They were having a great father–daughter bonding time when they came to the bottom of a long hill, and he unwisely challenged his daughter to see who would get to the top of the hill first. He won, but when his daughter reached the top of the run, her father was suffering sudden onset of speech difficulty and right-sided weakness from a stroke. So until you've built up your capacity, don't put yourself in competitive situations and let your pride get in the way of good health.

Another major admonition is not to steal time from sleeping to invest in physical activity. That is fool's gold. Instead, be absolutely determined to get enough sleep. See what else you may need to sacrifice if you need to generate time to increase your fitness quotient, but don't take from your sleep time. Alternatively, explore how you can integrate increased physical activity into your regular day, then bask in the glow of compliments people will make about how sharp your mind is!

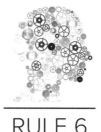

RULE 6

Sleep Enough ... If You Want to Think with Ease!

Life can get in the way of a good night's sleep. The demands of work and home can combine to impair our ability to get the amount of sleep we need. In nearly any city, rush hour can start at 5 a.m. and end at 9 p.m. Insufficient sleep has become so common that the U.S. Centers for Disease Control and Prevention are calling the current situation a public health epidemic. We all have known individuals who brag that they need little sleep to function well. Forget it. Most common mortals like you and me need a full night's sleep. Besides, people who cheat themselves of good sleep do not function well and are not thinking or performing cognitively at their full capacity.

We need sleep of good quality and of sufficient duration if we want our minds and our bodies to be alert and function optimally. For most people this means sleeping soundly for about eight hours. If your sleep is interrupted because you need to go to the bathroom frequently, or because there is activity in the house, or because you live next to a noisy airport or a busy highway, you may need to adjust that figure upwards.

A patient was sent to me recently because an emergency physician who saw her wanted to be sure she was not suffering from a seizure disorder. She was a very pleasant 52-year-old who told me she was driving to work at 8 a.m. and remembers thinking to herself, "The second right exit is mine." The next thing she knew she was in the left lane heading towards the ditch. She could not remember how she had gotten over to the left lane. She was so rattled that at work she kept shaking whenever she needed to write something, so she decided to call her husband to come and get her. She had a hard time remembering his phone number, which rattled her even more. He finally came and drove her to the emergency room. She was examined and her neurological test was found to be normal. A CT scan of the brain was ordered and she was referred for an electroencephalogram (EEG) to check for seizures and was referred to me. She was told she could not drive until her diagnosis was clarified and a note was sent to that effect to the appropriate motor vehicle department.

She was understandably upset at how upside down her life had suddenly become. I examined her and reviewed with her the results of lab tests. Her general physical and neurological examinations were normal, but cognitive testing revealed her to have diminished memory function. Her MoCA score was 24/30. Her brain CT scan showed atrophy too pronounced for her age, but no acute trouble like a stroke or a bleed. Her EEG did not reveal any seizure activity. After I conveyed these results to her, I started asking questions about her lifestyle, and I could not believe what I was hearing. This patient told me that she usually went to bed at midnight because she liked to watch a late TV show, got up at 5:30 a.m. to get ready for her work, and usually left the house around 7:30 a.m. She needed two hours in the morning to get herself ready, take her dog for a walk, and prepare breakfast for the family. I asked her about her sleep environment. She slept next to her husband and the dog shared their bed! Her husband snored, which made her sleep fitfully, and he got up to go to the bathroom twice a night to pee. Whenever he got up, the dog awakened and this awakened her. This patient was in bed a total of 5½ hours, with her sleep interrupted multiple times. She was embarrassed as she agreed with me that the most likely cause of her changing lanes without wanting to was that she had fallen asleep. She also confirmed that she had been suffering from forgetfulness that was affecting her efficiency at work. When I told her that driving with as little sleep as she had was akin to driving drunk and could be fatal, she agreed through her tears. These were my recommendations to her:

1. Go to bed at 9:30 p.m. if she needed to get up at 5:30 a.m. I suggested she record the late-night TV show for weekend viewing if it was that important, or avoid it altogether.

2. She should sleep in a separate bedroom, alone. Her husband should see his physician to see if he had sleep apnea.

3. Keep the dog off her bed and out of her room.

When I next saw her, she could not believe how much brighter her mind was, and how much her memory function and efficiency at work had improved. She was also slightly embarrassed to tell me that her colleagues at work had been complimenting her on her more pleasant personality and brighter outlook on life, which I gathered was quite an improvement on their previous assessment of her.

Why Is Sleep So Essential?

More studies are showing why sleep is so crucial to our physical and mental health. After all, every animal and human does it. If you think about it, throughout our human development, every time we went to sleep we were disconnected from our environment, and that put us at the mercy of whatever wild animal or danger was lurking around. That tells us that sleep must be essential if nature designed it that way. The brain is your most active organ and requires and consumes energy per unit weight that is multiples of any other organ in the body. Sleep is the opportunity for the brain to undergo a daily complete tune-up. It allows the brain the opportunity and time to wash away the exhaust material, the toxins that built up during the day's mental activities.[1] During sleep, brain repair is turned on, and the production of myelin is revved up—that is the white matter in the brain that facilitates rapid internal communication so essential for normal cognitive functions.[2] So sleep contributes to restoring brain function.

The Consequences of Sleep Deprivation on the Mind

When you go with less sleep than you need, in addition to feeling fatigue and being slow, every system in your body is negatively affected, particularly if sleep deprivation is prolonged. In chronic sleep deprivation, blood pressure goes up and stays up, hardening of the arteries is accelerated, and the risk of cardiovascular disease like heart attack and stroke is higher. It is also clear that when you have not slept enough, you don't possess the energy to be physically active, so over time those who are chronically tired are more likely to develop sedentary habits. They also tend not only to eat more but also choose high-energy foods that contain more fat.[3] Thus cheating your body of sleep is costly at all levels, and at all ages. A policy statement by the American Academy of Pediatrics emphasizes the need for sufficient sleep in children and adolescents and outlines the short- and long-term consequences of chronic sleep deprivation.[4]

Nor is the mind spared, as my patient's MoCA results showed. The brain uses sleep as an opportunity to repair connections that may have been damaged during the day and to consolidate learning that happened while we were awake. It is therefore not surprising that too little sleep reduces mental processes like learning, memory, judgement, and problem-solving. I referred to the CEO of the brain—the frontal lobes and their ability to direct attention to what is relevant. Sleep deprivation has a major detrimental effect on frontal lobe function and makes thinking very fuzzy, which some have likened to the cognitive impact of alcoholism.

Brain-imaging studies in individuals who chronically get less sleep than they need confirm what my patient's scan showed: loss of brain volume beyond what might be expected for the patient's age. Poor sleep quality or duration is associated with increased atrophy in the brain regions that serve our ability to have good judgement and clear reasoning and make sound decisions.[5] A study on the effect of sleep duration on thinking and brain structure showed that cheating on sleep duration accelerates brain shrinkage and causes a decline in cognitive performance. People who are well rested are better able to learn a task and more likely to remember what they learned.[6] Thus, lack of adequate sleep impairs our mental functions and aggravates the factors that tend to diminish them.

Another less recognized consequence of sleep deprivation is its impact on our psyche. When people are deprived of sleep, the first and most obvious impact is on their mood. Insomnia increases the risk of developing depression. Since one of the most important indicators of depression is insomnia and poor sleep quality, you can see the vicious cycle that sleep deprivation can induce. Sadness is exacerbated when we lie awake at night, unable to sleep. A study recently showed that just one hour less sleep during an entire week was associated with significantly greater odds of feeling hopeless, of substance abuse, and of suicidality.[7] This also works in reverse: getting good sleep is therapeutic and can lift depression. This bidirectional relationship between sleep and our mental health has been proven in recent studies showing that curing insomnia in depressed individuals significantly increases their chances of recovery from the depression.

Falling Asleep and Staying Asleep

Unfortunately, some people have trouble falling asleep and staying asleep. It is estimated that 1 in 3 Canadians and 70 million Americans have trouble falling asleep, sleep poorly when sleep finally arrives, and carry on in a sleep-deprived state day after day. Sleep is not a luxury, and quality sleep is an absolute necessity. So make a pact with yourself that you will give top priority to optimizing your sleep in both quality and quantity. Let's establish some rules that will help you sleep better:

1. Tell yourself you don't *have* to watch the late-night news or that late-night TV show. It takes discipline, but if you must get up at 7:00 a.m., be in bed by 10:30 p.m. Arrange your bedtime so that you go to bed 8.5 hours before you have to get up. This will give you at least the 8 hours you need, and once you have established a routine, stick to it.

2. Teenagers need more sleep than adults do. Their internal clock is delayed compared to adults'. Some jurisdictions have recognized this fact, so school start times have been shifted to later and this has resulted in substantial benefits, including reduced absenteeism, less aggressive behaviour, and improved academic performance.

3. Total darkness and quiet are required to fall asleep and stay asleep. Put up those light-blocking shades, and when you are ready for bed, turn off all electronic equipment and screens in the room. The email that comes in the middle of the night can wait for the morning. You'll be called on your telephone if it's an emergency. Consider setting up your electronic device to only receive calls. In a recent Australian study, over 70% of adolescents reported having two or more electronic devices in their bedroom at night, and a large percentage of them reported night-time use of cellphones, computers, and TV.[8] Another article reported that teenagers send numerous text messages at night after they get into bed. There is a clear association between night-time use of these devices and the delay in sleep/wake schedules, with its potential negative impact on health and educational outcomes.

4. If you sleep next to someone who snores, it's time for one of you to move to a different bedroom and for the snorer to consult a family doctor about the possibility of sleep apnea. High levels of noise, be it from a sleeping partner, a busy highway close by, or aircraft flyovers, will affect sleep quality by fragmenting it and increasing night-time restlessness.

5. You love your pets and think of them as family members, but please leave all pets out of your bedroom and certainly

out of your bed. You can shower them with love in the morning and before you go to bed. Their presence in your bedroom will disrupt your sleep.

6. No naps during the day. Nodding off at your desk will deprive you of a good night's sleep.

7. You may feel cold when you get into bed, but if you use heavy covers to get warm, you might wake up during the night because you are too warm and sweaty. So keep the room cool and don't cover yourself too heavily. Your body heat trapped under the cover will soon make you comfortable.

8. A modest amount of exercise before you go to bed (going up and down the stairs in your house two or three times) helps avoid "restless leg syndrome," which can interfere with sleep, but if you exercise too much just before turning in, your body may be too wound up to relax and let you sleep. Try to find your happy medium for pre-bed activity and stick to it.

9. Develop a bedtime ritual—a sequence of activities you do just before you get into bed. Your brain will get ready to fall asleep when you follow the same routine every night. It doesn't matter what it is so long as you select it and stick to it for six weeks so it becomes a habit (remember the six-week rule?). It might go like this: I put on my pj's, brush my teeth and floss them, wash my face, put on my heavy socks, check that the doors are locked, then get into bed. The sequence can include meditating, a prayer, or going to a peaceful place in your imagination. It is essential to maintain the order in which these activities are completed in a ritualistic fashion to give your brain the message that it is sleep time.

10. Once in bed, some people use a progressive muscle relaxation routine, starting with getting one foot totally relaxed by finding a happy position for it, then go to the other foot and get it totally relaxed, then one knee, then another, then one leg, etc. You must also remember to include your shoulder and neck muscles in that relaxation ritual. Returning nightly to that ritual will be a signal to your brain to go nighty-night.

11. No coffee after 4 p.m. If you are nursing a cold or treating an infection, remember that caffeine and other stimulating ingredients can be found in over-the-counter medications, so pay attention to what you are ingesting.

12. Avoid the temptation to take sleeping pills to help you with your insomnia. They are not only habit forming but have also been shown to impair memory function and are associated with a reduction in cognitive functions. Some individuals believe that 3 mg of melatonin taken as they are going to bed help them fall asleep, but this drug is also habit forming and in the long run not terribly useful because of its potential for negative side effects.

13. If you are having a late supper, avoid a large meal and do not consume too much alcohol. One glass of wine should be the limit of what you drink when it is close to bedtime.

14. If you fall asleep when you put your feet up to watch the late news, get up and go to bed. One patient told me he sits down to watch the late news only after he has brushed his teeth, flossed, and put his pj's on. That way if he starts dozing in front of the TV, he can crawl directly into bed. It isn't ideal, but it works for him!

These good habits often form the core of cognitive behavioural therapy to induce better sleep. Cognitive behavioural therapy has been proven to work for those who suffer from chronic insomnia—this kind of therapy requires a specially trained psychologist.

Recognize and Treat Sleep Apnea

Sleep apnea is now recognized as a major impediment to normal memory and cognitive functions. It is very important therefore to recognize the condition, in yourself or your partner, and treat it promptly.

Individuals who suffer from sleep apnea usually snore at night, and if a partner shares their bed, they may notice that the affected individual will suddenly stop snoring, hold his or her breath for several seconds, then take one deep breath, and resume snoring. Often in this interval they move around in the bed and change position, indicating that they have lightened up on their sleep and perhaps their brain even woke up, although they may not recollect later that they woke up during the night. Nonetheless, these individuals awaken several times during the night and have terrible sleep quality. To confirm the presence of sleep apnea, a sleep study is performed in a hospital where the individual is observed and the quality of sleep is assessed, along with other specific measures.

People who suffer from sleep apnea do not feel refreshed in the morning. They are tired, irritable, and sleepy, and may in fact nod off during a meeting or at their desk. We've referred to the brain's gluttony when it comes to energy. While we are asleep, the brain is working very hard and needs to be constantly supplied with well-oxygenated blood. This is why we have to continue breathing and our hearts continue pumping while we are sleeping. In some individuals, however, the interruption in the breathing that occurs with sleep apnea is often an indication that the important deep-sleep phase called rapid eye movement (REM) sleep has been interrupted. Much memory consolidation occurs in that phase of sleep, and several reports indicate that individuals suffering from sleep apnea show significant cognitive deficits, including dementia. Certain structures in the brains of these individuals, such as the limbic system and other structures important for memory function, actually shrink in size. Over time those who suffer from sleep apnea become cognitively impaired and have trouble with memory, judgement, and decision-making, confirming a study showing that fragmented sleep was associated with higher risk of developing dementia.[9]

Sleep apnea is also a risk factor for developing high blood pressure and diabetes, so it is not surprising that the condition increases the risk of stroke and of dementia. Poor sleep quality and duration are associated with the appearance of microinfarcts in the brain.[10] Sleep apnea is more likely to occur in obese individuals, those who smoke, and those who consume too much alcohol. So the first efforts at reducing sleep apnea should be directed at discontinuing and diminishing any of these contributing factors. A treatment for sleep apnea, which must be applied if the affected individual wishes to preserve memory function in the short term and avoid strokes and dementia in the long term, is called CPAP, which stands for Continuous Positive Airway Pressure. It consists of a mask that is connected to a small machine that provides the mild pressure created by constant air flow to keep the individual's airways open. That way, the sleeper is assured of a good level of oxygen. If a sleep study shows that you suffer from sleep apnea, the clinic staff will train you on the correct and comfortable way to use CPAP. Several of my patients with sleep apnea who went this route reported that they could not believe the positive difference it made in their lives. They felt more alive, lighter in their step, and brighter in their minds. Treating the apnea will delay the appearance of cognitive difficulties and dementia symptoms by as much as 10 years.[11]

The Stages of Sleep

When we fall asleep, our brain goes through defined stages. That's right: while you sleep, oblivious to the world, your brain is working hard, going through a predefined sequence of stages. It is important to know about these stages because if your sleep is interrupted, the impact on your cognitive functions will depend on when in this cycle you woke up.

You have probably noticed that when you have just fallen asleep, you wake up easily if, let's say, the phone rings. That's because you are in Stage 1 of your sleep cycle, defined by your eyes being still, not darting around. This Stage 1 sleep lasts a matter of short minutes, after which you go into Stage 2, when your body temperature goes down, you may feel cold if you do not have enough covers, and you are in what's called non–rapid-eye-movement (non-REM) sleep. The next phase is deep sleep, Stage 3, and is also non-REM. You're still not dreaming, but it is harder to wake you up. During this stage you will be oblivious to that phone if it rings, because your brain is too busy getting rid of the chemical detritus you accumulated during the day—this is an important stage for that reason. These three non-REM stages last altogether about 1.5 hours, and they are followed by the first relatively short REM cycle, called that because the eyes are darting rapidly from side to side. The entire sequence is then repeated, but with each repetition, the non-REM stages get shorter and the REM stage gets longer. Over the entire night, if we were to add up the time spent in each stage, we would probably conclude that an adult spends a quarter of the night in REM and the rest in non-REM, while a child may spend 50% of its sleep time in REM.

The longer we are asleep, the longer is the relative duration of REM during each successive stage. So if you miss that last cycle because you have to wake up sooner than eight hours of sleep have gone by, you are interrupting your longest REM phase, and you may have trouble remembering previous events. You will also feel groggy and slightly confused. And if this goes on night after night, cognitive trouble and dementia will be the outcome.

Several studies confirm that when we are asleep, we are processing life's events and consolidating recently acquired memories, converting them into long-term memories. So far it has not been possible to state categorically which sleep stage is more crucial for certain memories than another, but a recent review on the topic leaves no doubt about the crucial role sleep plays in memory consolidation.[12] So if your sleep is too short, or it gets interrupted, your memory will be weakened and your other cognitive functions will also be impaired.

So, in conclusion, don't cheat yourself of a good night's sleep.

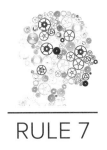

RULE 7

Socialize and Feel Useful: Loneliness and Depression Can Make You Crazy

We are programmed to interact socially and develop close emotional bonds with other people. A colleague used to say that human beings thrive only when they are sufficiently close to the important people in their lives: close enough emotionally to know their vulnerabilities, and close enough physically to smell their bad breath. Our mental health thrives when we can maximize the positive interactions and minimize those that leave us frustrated or sad. But we live in a world where individuals by and large just want to go about their business, improve their ability to acquire things, and are largely self-absorbed. At times it feels like all any of us can do is just hang in there. So it is often hard to break the mould and interact with other people in a meaningful way. But if meaningful social interaction, essential for our cognitive and emotional well-being, is not going to happen easily, it puts the burden on each one of us to try harder.

Each of us desperately needs the feeling of closeness—real human-to-human closeness. Having lots of friends on Facebook does not guarantee that we are not lonely. In my judgement, what matters is the emotional connection you have with people, especially those you have physically around you.

How Lonely Are We?

The statistics about loneliness in society are really disturbing. They suggest that many of us suffer from feeling lonely. In the United States, if you feel alone, you are in good company! In 2012, 27% of American households contained only one person, and it has been estimated that 40% of Americans feel lonely.[1] A survey by Statistics Canada in 2012 reported that 20% of older people in Canada declare feeling lonely.[2] And it gets worse for our youth: over a period of 12 months, two-thirds of university students reported feeling "very lonely." In Vancouver, a survey conducted by a charity found that one-third of all 25- to 34-year-olds were more alone than they liked.[3] These statistics are essentially double what they were 30 years ago.

The Causes of Social Isolation

If emotional closeness is one key to our cognitive health, what is interfering with our ability to form these emotional bonds?

1. *Economics.* Most of us are concerned with maximizing our own well-being, often forcing us to decrease our concern for others. To achieve economic success, we put up with a lot of dislocation, fighting rush-hour traffic, leaving home a lot, cheating ourselves out of sufficient sleep, all of which lead us to limit the time we could devote to others. In a

recent survey by the *Globe and Mail* newspaper, 60% of the 7,300 respondents reported feeling stressed and being unable to manage pressures of work and private lives. These individuals were more likely to overeat, drink alcohol, gamble, and be less productive at work.[4]

2. *Devalued loyalty.* We are in a society where loyalty is less and less a driver of our actions. No matter how long you have been in a relationship, a break-up is always a possibility and unfortunately can occur all too easily. Loyalty, be it to a life partner or an employer, is of diminished importance and value in current thinking, and relationships increasingly are victims of our self-absorbed society.

3. *The fractured family.* In my clinical experience, it has become too easy for a parent to tell their partner they are leaving the established partnership. In these break-ups, no matter how amicable they are, the children remain marked for the rest of their lives. Essentially they forever harbour the feeling that if they had been important enough, the couple would have stayed together. They lose confidence in the safety of their emotional and even physical environments, and prepare themselves for unforeseen and unpredictable emotional hits. They often become hypervigilant, which may translate into an anxiety syndrome and depression. Frequently these children become self-centred and recreate in later relationships the emotionally unpredictable environment they experienced earlier. I recognize, of course, that there are toxic relationships that are better for all concerned to be dissolved, and situations in which the children have to be removed from abusive environments, but these are far fewer than there are break-ups. Importantly, there have been many studies showing that

women who had to cope with major emotionally laden personal events such as divorce or unexpected bereavement were more likely to suffer serious physical ailments like heart attacks and also were more at risk to suffer from dementia later.[5]

4. *City dwelling, and specifically condo dwelling.* Forty percent of high-rise dwellers feel lonely compared to 22% of those living in detached homes, because the sense of community and neighbourliness is much reduced in the condo setting.

5. *Digital connectivity.* A major factor that distinguishes everyone's life from previous generations is the pervasive presence of electronic devices. While these devices are undoubtedly very useful, they do have an impact in various ways. First, because using most electronic devices usually demands that we stand still or sit, the excessive sedentary existence that is imposed on us by these devices has consequences already described. As well, sedentary behaviour in children has been associated with slower brain development and lower feelings of self-worth and self-esteem. Second, ideal interactions with parents, family members, and friends are physical and emotional. People who walk while using their electronic device are not interacting with their human and physical environments and they are reducing any positive impact that comes from those interactions. Children have complained that their parents must find them boring since the parents are always on their electronic devices rather than interacting with them. Our "friends" in many cases are connected to us only through the electronic medium, and while texting and other means of modern social interaction are perhaps

better than isolated silence, they are not as satisfying as face-to-face contacts. A recent study suggested that using Facebook increases the sense of loneliness.[6] Facebook friends are not there to hug you when you are sad and can't help you move a piece of furniture around in your room. You would think that social media would offer an opportunity for increased human connectivity, but in fact it accentuates the sense of loneliness because everyone else hypes the good times they are reporting, and everyone except you seems to be having fun. Finally, in some cases, access to the Internet and social media can have all the characteristics of an addiction: there is internal pressure to connect, even at the cost of rest or sleep, and doing so provides a quick fix.

We have to admit that we have the world that we have! We can wish it were different, but it is now structured to increase our sense of being alone. If individually and collectively we do not do something to regain our emotionally meaningful social networks, there are consequences that are already evident, and there is more to come.

Impact of Social Isolation and Loneliness on Our Health

Social bonds are crucial to our health, and social contact, especially if pleasant, has all kinds of benefits. Think of it. What happens in your brain when you are with people you like? First, before you even meet with your social partner, you are probably looking forward to the event and are excited about it. You may recall happy times that you shared in the past. Then when you first see your social partner, your brain's centres for face recognition are activated, and you greet your friend by first name, again requiring an activation of more brain memory centres. When you share memories with your friend, receive advice on daily life, and chat about different issues, that requires you to keep alert and activate your brain's cognitive and emotional centres. If during the conversation you touch hands or tap shoulders, or if you hug at the beginning or the end of the meeting, that human contact activates hormones such as oxytocin, which results in lowering stress levels and blood pressure. No wonder oxytocin is called the "cuddle hormone." So social activity and the sense of social and emotional connectedness activate the brain in positive ways. As well, good feelings lead to a decline in the activity of stress hormones and the inflammatory immune system, and that protects your blood vessels and brain.

It is therefore not surprising that several studies have concluded that individuals who are socially active seem not only to extend their lives in years, but also appear to be protected from cognitive decline as they age. Their memory functions are better, and their brain scans look a lot younger than their chronological age.[7] A 2014 Dutch study showed that feeling lonely was associated with a 64% increase in the risk of developing dementia.[8]

In addition to dementia, loneliness is associated with a number of health consequences. First, there is the increasing likelihood of obesity. Food becomes the only sure source of pleasure, and lonely people suffer a tendency to consume high-calorie items. Feeling alone also increases the likelihood of depression, augments aggressiveness towards others, and heightens the risk of suicide. The feeling of loneliness also suppresses our immune system, making us more liable to get infections, increases our sense of fatigue, and accelerates the hardening of our arteries, making it more likely that we suffer heart attacks and strokes. Loneliness even raises the likelihood of suffering from cancer. So that sense of being alone in a world that doesn't care about you, if persistent, leads to a whole lot of physical and emotional trouble. Perhaps for all these reasons, one researcher reported that people who say they are socially isolated and lonely increase their chances of dying by 30% compared to those who did not express such negative emotions.[9]

Let me not mince words: Having really good friends and a close family network and interacting with people you know genuinely care about you contribute to a longer and happier life and one where cognitive function is more likely to be preserved and dementia more likely to be kept at bay.

How to Avoid Social Isolation

People have gone to great lengths to avoid loneliness. Here are some examples:

1. *Postponing retirement.* I will grant you that having a job does not guarantee a sense of usefulness. A recent U.K.study reported a correlation between being bored at work and the development of cardiac risk factors.[10] So when we say someone is "bored to death," it may not be too far-fetched. In a successful work environment, we feel connected to those we work with. This may well be why so many of us are reluctant to retire. Going to work, painful as it is sometimes, does provide us with an intellectual and social environment that is healthy, assuming work is not accompanied by adverse professional and social impacts. Work makes most of us feel useful. It validates our efforts. A recent study from France reviewed

the records of more than 400,000 workers, most of them shopkeepers or craftsmen who had some control over their retirement age, and compared their health information to those who had to retire by virtue of their work contract. The study concluded that the risk of dementia was lowered by 3.2% for each year that retirement was postponed after the age of 60.[11] This may be why retirement is on the decline. A recent survey by the U.S. Bureau of Labour Statistics showed that 18.7% of Americans older than 65 remained at work, a 34% increase from a decade ago, and 20.1% of those between the ages of 70 and 74 did the same.[12]

2. This is not an exhortation to work till death. It is only to emphasize that you should not go from an active, structured, and intellectually and socially rewarding life at work to a social and intellectual vacuum after retirement. Take it from Sister Constance Murphy, a Canadian Anglican nun and gerontologist who died in 2013 while still active at the age of 109. She believed that the most important thing senior citizens can do was to try new things and stay active—physically, mentally, and spiritually.[13] She added: "Second or even third careers can be taken up by old people, through volunteer work or through higher education." So if you are going to retire, make absolutely certain to create opportunities for yourself to lead a structured existence, rich with intellectual stimulation, and socially rewarding. Make sure before you retire that you have a clear plan of how, post-retirement, you will find opportunities to validate your existence in the world and your value to society. You can find positive fulfilling work between the end of your career and full retirement.

3. *Volunteering.* A recent paper in *Psychological Bulletin* reviewed all the evidence on the benefits of volunteering.[14] It confirmed that volunteering reduced symptoms of depression, improved overall health, and conferred longevity. Interestingly, the authors found that the "sweet spot" for the level of volunteering that accomplishes these good outcomes was two to three hours a week. So volunteering need not be too demanding to provide its benefits.

4. *Seeking fleeting contact.* If social activities are not pursued, some individuals report going for body massages just to feel human contact. A freelance writer was reported to have switched to being a waitress just to have more human contact.[15] Prostitutes will tell you many of their customers are hungrier for the human emotional contact than the sexual activity. Some organizations have recognized this social need and offer settings for random hugs given to anyone who will come forward.

5. *Adopting a pet.* I believe the explosion in the number of pets we have in Western societies coincides with urbanization and its consequent aggravation of our sense of loneliness. In Canada, the total human population is less than 40 million, but we own 26 million pets: 38% of households have a cat, and 35% have a dog. And here is the best statistic: 80% of individuals who have a pet consider them to be family. Pets decrease our sense of being alone in the world, so even though our cities are spread out with no central meeting places or green spaces, and our closest loved ones may be an airplane ride away, many of us have got pets just so some living creature is happy to see us when we show up, predictably and reliably, and makes us feel happier and less alone.

Loneliness Can Morph into Depression

Being surrounded by people does not protect you from feeling lonely if you don't feel that they care about you enough. Feeling lonely is an inner feeling of "I don't matter, and if I wasn't here I would not be missed much." It can result in anxiety, depression, and hostility towards others.

Let's face it, some interactions are best avoided. If a so-called friend or a relative gives you hell every time they see you, and the interaction is unpleasant and makes you stressed, you don't need people like that in your life. If interacting with a particular individual is anxiety-provoking and unpleasant, warn them once or twice, but if they persist, stop seeing them. Negative social interactions are detrimental to our cognitive capacities.

Having said that, it is important to emphasize that if we are to avoid depression, loneliness has to be actively resisted. The state of depression is fraught with all kinds of physical consequences. In the state of depression the likelihood of diabetes, heart attacks, strokes, and premature aging are all increased.[16] These conditions in turn make depression more likely, resulting in a classic positive feedback process, or vicious cycle. As stated, there is an increased risk of heart attacks and strokes after bereavement or divorce, and these conditions raise the risk of dementia. For these reasons, one researcher believes loneliness and social isolation should be taken seriously as threats to public health.[17]

It is also important to note that taking antidepressants does not seem to reduce the physical and cognitive consequences of depression. Over a four-year period from 1992 to 1996, the rate of office-based visits in which a diagnosis of depression was made and antidepressants prescribed in the United States increased 18.5% for whites, 38.5% for blacks, and 106.7% for Hispanics.[18] Although a lot of us are taking antidepressants and these medications reduce the feelings of sadness, they don't seem to calm the inflammation that has been revved up in the body by the depression.

You can see it is important to find social and emotional ways to effectively reduce the likelihood of loneliness turning into depression, and the remedy against loneliness, regardless of your circumstances, is to develop a sense of your own value to yourself and to your environment.

At the practical level, anything you can do to feel you are contributing to the well-being of others will be a step away from loneliness and depression and a step towards your own well-being. Those actions will generate and sustain the feeling that you do matter. Let me give you some examples that have been reported recently:

- ▸ The doorman. A young high school student who had been bullied and was depressed invented a service. He gained self-confidence and a sense of self-worth simply by holding doors open to other students and passers-by. He received special recognition for the service, it made him feel useful, and everyone else appreciated the act.

- ▸ The growth in community gardens. Neglected parcels of land are getting transformed into gardens, bringing neighbours together to share a productive outdoor activity while socially engaged.

- ▸ Community events that bring people together have included knitting circles, pumpkin-carving competitions, cooking lessons, origami workshops, highland dancing, get-togethers such as ceilidhs, and mall-walking groups. This last one is my favourite because it combines a physical activity with social interaction.

▸ Hugs and cuddles for sale. Yup! The realisation that many of us are deprived of human contact and that human touch has enormous physical and psychological benefits has led to hugging and cuddling as a service you can pay for.

When you review the activities suggested here, the common thread through them is that you are with people, you are in a social setting that is safe and pleasant, and the activity results in you feeling involved and useful. The more the activity is undertaken in nature, and the more it involves people, the more likely it is to alleviate loneliness. So smile at your neighbours, and surprise them by performing an unexpected kindness towards them. Making yourself useful to others and contributing to their well-being, even if you have to invent a service, is the key to warding off loneliness. When you've participated in some of these activities, stand in front of your mirror, and smile a heart-felt genuine smile approvingly at yourself.

Volunteering for good causes also provides a sense of usefulness in our community and social environment. There is no end to the opportunities to volunteer your time, your energy, your advice, your professional skills, your wisdom, and the lessons you learned in life that you can pass on. Bring a smile to someone, volunteer to feed the hungry, contribute to the welfare of a younger person, and offer your professional services gratis. You will be the biggest beneficiary.

Can I Test Whether I Am Depressed?

A questionnaire has been developed to help you and your physician assess the presence and severity of your depression. It is called the Patient Health Questionnaire (PHQ-9)—see Table 4. The questionnaire can be used for screening, diagnosing, measuring, and monitoring the severity of depression. The value of this tool has been tested and is proven.[19]

TABLE 4

Patient Health Questionnaire				
Patient name:				
Date of visit:				
Over the past 2 weeks, how often have you been bothered by any of the following problems?	Not at All	Several Days	More Than Half of the Days	Nearly Every Day
Little interest or pleasure in doing things?	0	1	2	3
Feeling down, depressed, or hopeless?	0	1	2	3
Trouble falling asleep, staying asleep, or sleeping too much?	0	1	2	3
Feeling tired or having little energy?	0	1	2	3
Poor appetite or overeating?	0	1	2	3
Feeling bad about yourself—or that you're a failure or have let yourself or your family down?	0	1	2	3
Trouble concentrating on things, such as reading the newspaper or watching television?	0	1	2	3

continued...

TABLE 4

Patient Health Questionnaire				
Over the past 2 weeks, how often have you been bothered by any of the following problems?	Not at All	Several Days	More Than Half of the Days	Nearly Every Day
Moving or speaking so slowly that other people have noticed? Or, the opposite— being so fidgety or restless that you have been moving around a lot more than usual?	0	1	2	3
Thoughts that you would be better off dead or of hurting yourself in some way?	0	1	2	3
TOTAL	0	9	18	27

If you checked off any problems, how difficult have those problems made it for you to do your work, take care of things at home, or get along with other people?

☐	☐	☐	☐
Not difficult at all	Somewhat difficult	Very difficult	Extremely difficult

The questions are answered by grading the severity of the responses. The total PHQ-9 score is then used to provide both a provisional diagnosis and treatment recommendations as follows (see Table 5):

TABLE 5

Scoring the PHQ-9		
PHQ SCORE	**PROVISIONAL DIAGNOSIS**	**TREATMENT RECOMMENDATION**
0 to 4	Not depressed	
5 to 9	Minimal symptoms*	Support, educate to call if worse, return in 1 month
10 to 14	Minor depression++ Dysthymia * Major depression, mild	Support Antidepressant or psychotherapy Antidepressant or psychotherapy
15 to 19	Major depression, moderately severe	Antidepressant or psychotherapy
≥ 20	Major depression, severe	Antidepressant and psychotherapy (especially if not improved on monotherapy)

If symptoms are present for ≥ two years, then the probability of chronic depression that warrants antidepressants or psychotherapy is high.

++ If symptoms present ≥ one month or severe functional impairment is present, consider active treatment.

Social Connections Using Computers and Hand-held Devices

It is not enough to be connected only through social media! I have already covered some of the problems with electronic connections, but it is worth stating again that there is growing recognition that communicating through the computer medium is a double-edged sword. If you use it to Skype or use other media to connect with someone face to face on the screen, it is better than silence and isolation, but the sense of being connected is fleeting and somewhat devoid of reality. It is not as emotionally satisfying as sitting with someone you like to converse and interact with. You can't reach through the screen and hug the person you're talking to.

Texting or other messaging mediums are also emotionally stunted. It is so much richer for our mind and healthier for our psyche to gauge someone else's moods, recognize their facial expressions and the tone of their voice, watch their body language, predict their reactions to what we are saying, and if appropriate have some kind of physical contact. When the connection is by email or texting, it is difficult to judge the tone of a text message, decide what the sender's state of mind is, and divine their facial expression or mood. As a result, if we use technology as our predominant means of contact with the outside world, many parts of our brains are not activated. Electronic contact may be preferable to no contact, but it is a very limited and limiting medium from a cognitive standpoint.

Research literature is increasingly commenting on the health consequences of being in the hypervigilant state that our computers and hand-held devices keep us in for all our waking, and frequently also sleeping, hours. We were designed to be hypervigilant only for short bouts of time, when we met foes or beasts, not for hours at a time. Consequently, hyper-tension and rapid heart rates are being reported in individuals who cannot disconnect from their email stacks, which of course rebuild as soon as you triage through them! Being disconnected from our environment while we are doing email and texting for hours has even been reported to result in an IQ drop. For all these reasons, companies that value their employees' well-being are starting to encourage them to disconnect when they are not at work, even going as far as shutting their server down in the evenings.

This issue of connectedness is likely worse if you are young and grew up with computers from your early days. Americans over the age of 65 are devoting 6 hours and 40 minutes a day to socializing, relaxing, and leisure, but that activity rapidly decreases with younger ages.[20] In fact there is now a lot of concern about the potential cognitive impact of our children's obsession with screens and devices. One grandfather exclaimed: "There is no conversation anymore. When the family dines out, the boys use their devices before the meal arrives and as soon as they finish eating. They have no interest in learning from our experiences, no time to daydream, and no interest in sharing their thoughts or anxieties with their parents."

What Not Do When You Feel Alone

Here are some activities—or non-activities!—to avoid when you feel alone.

▶ When feeling alone, falling into the trap of increasing time in front of the TV can be toxic. It can lead to the conversion of being alone into feeling lonely—and that transition should be avoided. Whatever else you do, don't turn on the TV because you are bored. TV viewing is one-way communication that does not stimulate the brain sufficiently, and to make matters worse, most people watch TV sitting and boredom is often remedied by eating. That is a triple whammy that contradicts many of the rules in this book. Don't do it.

▶ To reiterate the points made earlier about the potential health consequences of being connected by email day and night, there is growing consensus that we need to turn our electronic devices off to reconnect with our natural, social, and emotional environments. I strongly recommend that you turn off all your computer devices at night. Do not use your smartphone to check the time if you wake up during night so you are not tempted to check emails. If you think you're getting extra brownie points because you send work-related emails in the dead of night, you are paying for it with your health.

▶ Another admonition is not to go to a bar. Merrymaking fuelled by booze will soon fade and send you to the opposite extreme. Socializing contributes to our sense of well-being, and enhances our cognitive abilities, but it has to be done the right way, and going to a bar is not it.

If you suffer through prolonged periods of feeling that you are your only friend, and that others do not care about your well-being, the consequences may include the development of a short temper; lashing out at colleagues; seeking reliable and predictable pleasures such as overeating, drinking, or drug addiction; or a combination of these. If you stay indoors, avoid social activities, and don't develop a sense of usefulness to people around you, you are succumbing to your loneliness and it is likely that it will morph into depression, with its enormous consequences to the health of your brain and mind.

Depression Can Lead to Dementia
I have gone into detail on how to avoid loneliness that can morph into depression because the medical literature is now

very clear: depression when prolonged contributes to dementia. In a recent systematic review of the factors associated with cognitive decline in later life, researchers looked at all large observational studies and randomized controlled trials published over 25 years. They concluded there was an association between depression and the development of dementia, thus confirming a growing consensus.[21] In fact, other researchers reported that half of the patients with major depressive disorders exhibited generalized thinking and memory impairment.[22]

Depression seems to bring about changes in our body that favour many of the risk factors associated with dementia and that you are by now familiar with. First, depression seems to accelerate the process of aging. Scientists can look at any cell in our body and measure the length of a region called the telomere that appears at the ends of a chromosome. From that they can determine your biological age: not necessarily your age in years, but the extent of wear and tear in your cells that indicate biological age. When scientists in the Netherlands did that recently, they found that people who were or had been depressed had shorter telomeres, meaning their bodies had aged more rapidly, even when all other factors were taken into account.[23] So depression will add to your age years you have not lived.

Depression is also a big a risk factor for small strokes. It is as big a risk as high blood pressure.[24] A recent imaging study has found that depressed individuals show abnormalities in the same brain regions known to be vulnerable to the development of the small covert white matter strokes we referred to earlier.[25] This came as a shock to me when I first learned of it. I was quite familiar with the reverse, namely that those individuals who were unfortunate enough to have suffered a stroke became subsequently depressed, but the fact that depression made strokes more likely was not emphasized in the medical literature until recently. So depression leads to muddled thinking and weakens memory functions by increasing the likelihood of the small strokes that occur in the brain's white matter. These new findings point to the vicious cycle of depression leading to small strokes, which worsen the depression, causing both dementia and more strokes to occur. It is thus extremely important to avoid depression if we want to spare our mind.

Why Should Depression Cause Strokes?

Depression seems to increase the likelihood of stroke through a number of mechanisms that work together to cause brain damage. I have tried to show all these elements in Figure 10 (it originally appeared in an article I wrote that appeared in *Cardiovascular Psychiatry and Neurology* in 2011).[26] It shows the mechanisms by which depression damages our brain, leading to dementia.

First of all, our heart and blood vessels respond to our state of mind. When the impact of emotions on the function of heart and blood vessels was studied, sadness was shown to result in a distinct pattern, with moderate increases in blood pressure and vascular resistance, and a decrease in the heart's pumping capacity.[27] If these responses persist in a person whose sadness does not lift, and he or she becomes chronically depressed, they will cause injury to the brain.

Our body interprets depression as constant stress. In April 2013 Dutch scientists published a study in which they analyzed accumulated cortisol levels in hair as an index of the persistence of stress. They found that those with high levels of cortisol in their hair had a much higher incidence of vascular

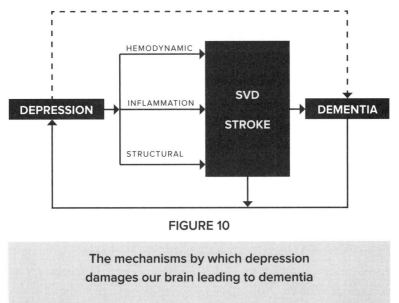

FIGURE 10

The mechanisms by which depression damages our brain leading to dementia

This vicious cycle leads to dementia, which in turn accentuates the entire cycle. SVD refers to small vessel disease strokes. The dotted line represents other mechanisms that may cause dementia related to depression.

disease and diabetes.[28] So persistent depression will age our blood vessels.

Depression also undermines our ability to regulate our appetites and increases our tendency for risky behaviour such as smoking or drinking. As social neuroscientist John Cacioppo, who with co-author William Patrick wrote a book titled *Loneliness: Human Nature and the Need for Social Connection*, says, "We want to soothe the pain we feel by maintaining high levels of sugar and fat delivered to the pleasure centers of the brain." So depression can also lead to obesity, another hit against our vascular and mental health.

Potentially the most relevant mechanism linking depression to both strokes and cognitive decline is the response of our immune system to sustained depression. It seems that when we are depressed our body reacts as if we have been chronically invaded by a bad virus or suffer from an incurable illness. Molecules are produced that can lead to strong inflammation in the body. Several studies have reported that compounds we refer to as inflammatory cytokines are increased in the bloodstream of depressed patients.[29] These same agents are known to damage the lining of the blood vessels and eventually lead to their narrowing through accelerated atherosclerosis. Thus depression causes the same kind of damage to our blood vessels that we see with smoking, obesity, and the aging process, all of which are associated with a chronic low-grade increase in inflammatory cytokines. This suggests that depression can accentuate the vascular-damaging effects of other conditions, and all this damage leads to dementia.[30]

How to Avoid Depression

I've referred to activities you should avoid when you are feeling lonely in order not to exacerbate the condition. There is another side to that coin, namely activities you can pursue that may lessen your lonely feelings and lighten your depression.

Bring Music Into Your Life

1. Listen to music you enjoy! Music activates many parts of our brain and mind. Many have written extensively about this, but especially my colleague Robert Zatorre, who has studied how musical perception leads to pleasure.[31] If the music you listen to gives you pleasure, it is cognitively useful to your brain. Music gives your brain a workout by activating many brain centres and connections. In chronic stroke patients, music that is perceived by the brain as pleasurable improves the plasticity of the brain and enhances recovery.[32]

It has been shown that musicians with at least 10 years of instrumental musical training remain cognitively sharp in advanced age,[33] and a report presented at the European Society of Cardiology showed that those who listened to their favourite music for just 30 minutes a day improved their exercise ability by 19%.[34] Melodies you love make you more fit—without increasing exercising! And here is further evidence of the power of music: it is a major way to build cognitive reserve. Many articles emphasize the emotional and cognitive benefits of regular musical activity even when cognitive decline has started.[35] We still don't know all the health-promoting mechanisms that music activates, but it is clear that listening to music you enjoy enhances cognition even as you age.

2. Better still, put on some music and move your butt to it! Get up and step to the music! Go dancing if you can! I have always thought that dancing should be part of our post-retirement activities. It combines listening to music with moving your body to a rhythm and provides social interaction. I have noticed recently that some churches are opening their basements to evenings of dancing for the parishioners. That's great use of space that sits otherwise mostly idle, and the activity brings together people to socialize in a pleasant ambiance. The tradition of ceilidhs, common in the Maritimes and Scotland, are worth introducing across the country. Snacks are usually provided, along with nice music by a live band. Many people go just to be engaging in social interaction, but when I'm at a ceilidh, I always feel like standing up and moving around, and maybe inviting a lady to dance. Ceilidhs are an opportunity to ward off dementia.

Several people have told me that square dancing wards off dementia. There is no scientific evidence for this that I am aware of, but the proponents point out that square dancing activates many brain and body functions since the dancers have to listen to instructions, change their movements accordingly, keep in rhythm with their companions, move their limbs in unison, all while they are enjoying music and companionship. They may be onto something. The Depressed Adolescents Treated with Exercise (DATE) study showed that in 12- to 18-year-olds, exercise can be an effective non-medication intervention in adolescents with major depressive disorder.[36] So if square dancing is for you, go for it.

3. Join a choir if you can. Being in a choir is like having group music therapy, with the added benefit of the social connections that form among choir members and the sense that you are giving pleasure to others—all in one shot. It alleviates depression and enhances thinking ability and memory functions.[37]

Take Noise Out

Many of us carry a set of earplugs, and others wear noise-cancelling earphones. Music has to speak to your inner being, and if you are forced to listen to music you don't like, it is potentially toxic to your mood and, if persistent, to your brain. Whether we are in a store or a restaurant or the elevator, we are often forced to listen to music that is not of our choice or our liking, and that's when earplugs come in handy.

If you are forced to listen to music you don't like, you are being exposed to noise. Our vascular system takes a direct hit with noise because it isn't designed to react to it. If it is hot outside, we sweat and that cools us down. If it is cold outside, our blood vessels relax to bring in more warm blood to our vital organs. The body has no similar physiological response to reduce noise. Noise is always interpreted by the body as an external threat.

There is now substantial literature on the negative impact of noise. Noise from airports has been linked to increased heart disease risk.[38] When people live close to airports, even though they claim not to be bothered by the noise, their vascular system nonetheless reacts negatively to it. And even if they remain asleep during the noise, they experience blood pressure spikes, and these ominous cardiovascular signals can persist.[39]

So minimize your exposure to noise, listen to a lot of music you enjoy, and while you do, get up and do a few dance steps!

Indulge Your Artistic Tendencies

When some of us were putting together the Canadian Stroke Network, we held a symposium dedicated to individuals who had suffered a stroke and invited them to come with their caregivers. One patient had the excellent idea of bringing in her paintings. She had been an amateur painter before she suffered a stroke and continued painting after her stroke. Most of the paintings were of flowers in a vase, and the sequence of paintings was fascinating. Prior to her stroke, the flowers in the vase were alive with colour, and the decorations on the vases were vibrant. After the stroke, the early paintings showed flowers that were outlined in a rudimentary way, and the most prevalent colours were blue, grey, and black. As the patient recovered, more colours crept into her painting, and the outlines became more defined. You could gauge the patient's struggles with the stroke and her gradual recovery of function just by looking at the sequence of her paintings.

Artistic indulgence is very stimulating to the brain and activates its memory centres. Confirmatory stories have sprung up on YouTube and documentary films as a testament to the fact that patients' imaginations are strengthened through artistic activities. So if you possess any artistic interests, indulge in them regardless of the degree of talent you may possess.

If the Depression Is Treated, Is the Associated Dementia Avoided?

If the depression is treated, additional damage to the brain is avoided, but the cognitive difficulties already suffered seem to go away only through the slow process of wilful recovery. So ideally, we should be alert and in touch with our feelings. Feelings such as sadness, anxiety, irritability, unrelenting stress, and not being useful to our social and family environments suggest that we may be heading towards depression. We should especially pay attention if these feelings are followed by physical symptoms such as fatigue, insomnia, lack of appetite, and headaches, indicating that the depression is upon us. It is important to act at that point, and act rapidly, to alleviate these feelings so that the awful consequences to our body and our brain referred to earlier can be avoided.

If despite everything you do to alleviate the symptoms the depression is unrelenting, it is imperative to seek medical and psychiatric attention. Psychotherapy, mindfulness training, and cognitive behavioural therapy have all been proven effective in alleviating depression. It is often important to treat the depression medically in addition to the psychotherapy, a path taken by many. Statistics show a significant rise in the use of antidepressants among all ethnic groups in the United States. In one province in Canada, antidepressant prescriptions dispensed to the 15 to 19 age group grew 10-fold in the 24-year period ending in 2007. While this suggests both increased awareness about the issue of depression and the rate of treating it, antidepressant medications do have side effects, and combining them with positive action such as I described in this chapter is often the only strategy that can provide long-term control of this condition.

Summary

Dementia is not inevitable as we get older. While it is ideal to start in our youth to enhance our brain's cognitive capacity, it is never too late.

There are positive influences on our brain's thinking and memory functions we need to bring about. That is the essence of Rule 1 in this book: use memory exercises, vary them, and keep your mind active.

We also need to avoid a number of negative influences. Above all, we must avoid impairing our brain with vascular disease. This means avoiding damaging our brain with strokes, both the kind we feel—which are treatable if attended to quickly—and the covert ones we may not feel. Both are damaging to our cognitive ability (Rule 2). As the major vascular risk that can lead to strokes and harm our brain is high blood pressure, it is imperative that we measure and record our blood pressure, aiming for 120/80 (Rule 3). A major and prevalent dementia risk factor is obesity, which in addition to being a pro-inflammatory state raises blood pressure and in its own right impairs cognition in the long run. Thus we need to eat right and weigh light in order to stay bright (Rule 4). The book provides solid advice on how to achieve this.

We have also learned recently that moderate exercise enhances our memory functions, and so advice is given on the kind and amount of exercise needed to keep our minds sharp (Rule 5).

The brain weighs only 2% of our body weight but consumes 20% of its entire energy output. Sleep is used by the body to clear the brain of the exhaust material accumulated by this revved-up engine, hence the need to sleep adequately (Rule 6), and we've examined how to enhance sleep duration and quality. Finally, the book strongly recommends keeping a bright spirit and avoiding sadness, loneliness, and depression, as these conditions encourage vascular disease, lead to strokes, and impair memory (Rule 7).

Epilogue

A Message to All Citizens, Especially Parents, Caregivers, Health Care Providers, Educators, and Governments

I hope reading this book has convinced you that you can do a lot yourself not only to preserve but even enhance your ability to think, your memory functions, your judgement, and your happiness quotient. The brain's commitment to dementia is made much earlier than the appearance of symptoms of cognitive trouble. If a person has inherited the gene for Alzheimer's disease, the script for dementia is already written by the time they are born, but as this book emphasizes, that is a relatively small minority of individuals who develop dementia, and even then, there is benefit to controlling and reducing the vascular risk to the brain. For most of us, the script determining whether we will become demented starts to be written in childhood and is close to completion by the middle years.

This does not mean that you should give up. Regardless of age, developing the right approaches and habits will diminish the chances of becoming cognitively impaired. That is why this book was written: there is always hope to avoid or moderate dementia. The brain registers and responds to everything that happens to us. It reacts to everything we do and everything we do not do with our bodies and our minds. So it is important to categorically state that we need a new personal and social contract to decrease the incidence and impact of dementia on individuals and on society.

It is crucial that we start by monitoring maternal health and protecting it if we are to avoid lifelong misery to the child, a heavy burden on the caring family, and major cost to our health care system. Supporting parents during their children's early years while they provide them with a physical, social, and intellectual environment that will enhance their cognitive functions is an important investment, not a cost.

These considerations have a major impact on the development of risk factors for dementia. I have outlined the statistics showing the increase in the prevalence of hypertension and obesity in young age groups. A Swedish study followed almost half a million men conscripted for military service over 37 years, during which some developed dementia.[1] High blood pressure in youth and excessive alcohol intake were strongly associated with the subsequent development of dementia. As well, associations of dementia with insufficient early education, sedentary lifestyle, and smoking were all confirmed in this study and restated in this book. For this reason, all those involved in the welfare of our youth—parents, daycare workers, educators, those determining school policies, school cafeteria managers, and those holding the public purse—need to be reminded that what we are exposed to throughout our life, but especially in the early and middle periods, has an impact on our subsequent mental health.

A word of warning is timely here. I have no doubt that some of you, convinced of the value in following the recommendations made in this book, will try to bring these changes into your lives. If you make some progress then give up, you may become hesitant to start over for fear of failure. Do not despair.

Changes as significant as the ones I have recommended in this book are not easy to implement. Remember that change can come about after several trials that were only partially successful. Some of my psychology colleagues tell me that when we attempt major changes in our lives, four to seven attempts may be necessary, on average, before success is finally achieved. So take heart!

If you have in the past tried to bring some of these changes into your life and failed, take pride in the fact that you have tried, and do not despair of ultimate success. Don't forget: "It is better to have tried and failed than never to have tried at all." After you have congratulated yourself for trying, change your past attempt into a learning experience. Why did the attempt fail? Was it because you were not totally convinced of the need for action? If reading this book has convinced you of the need to change and reignited your determination, let's make sure the components for success are all there:

1. You perceive in your heart of hearts the need to change one or more of the risk factors for dementia discussed in this book. You know the importance of doing this and have contemplated this move for a while and tried to change things before, with some success but no long-term impact. Don't be discouraged. Ask yourself if you are truly ready this time. If so, combine your personal motivation with changes you bring about in your environment.

2. Don't keep the decision to yourself. Share it with close friends, a life partner, and individuals you know care about your well-being. Being surrounded by empathy is important, so make sure you have in place the social support systems of friends and family who will be there to encourage you and cheer on your early successes.

3. You are more likely to succeed if you change the environment. A colleague decided she needed to lose weight and over the following year lost 47 pounds, the goal she had set for herself. She did it by changing her shopping habits. She knew that her major problem was frequent snacking after supper, usually with chips, sweets, or cookies. So she stopped shopping weekly and putting lots of food in her fridge. Instead, on the way home she would buy the healthy food items she was going to consume that day. Her cupboards at home were empty, and her fridge contained only the bare essentials. The food wasn't there, so she could not gorge herself. This new habit was not efficient, but she didn't give up because as she began to lose weight, her friends and colleagues were full of compliments, which reinforced her behaviour, hence her ultimate success.

Clearly, the example here goes counter to society's goal of making our lives easier and more time-efficient. One of this book's important tenets is to go counter to this trend: make your day harder and physically more demanding. It will take a bit more time, but it is time well-invested in your healthy future.

4. Take up the many challenges of modifying your lifestyle as suggested in this book, but do it one at a time. Attempting to monitor your blood pressure weekly, lose weight, increase physical activity, stop smoking, and follow the other advice in this book cannot be accomplished all at the same time. Conquer your demons one by one.

5. Celebrate small successes. Take pride in them and let them energize you to go on with the program suggested in this book. The goal of protecting your memory functions and your thinking abilities is worth it.

A Message to Parents

Since many of the factors that determine later dementia start in childhood, parents must assume a growing responsibility to influence behaviour before the teenage years. We visited a friend in his summer cottage recently. He and his wife were there with their toddler grandchild. The grandmother, my friend's wife, was feeding the child, who was in her baby chair. Supper was a cut-up hot dog that the child was gobbling down, and yes, the child appeared obese. I bit my tongue but was very disappointed. The opportunity for this grandmother to be a force for good was wasted. We must always remember that foods we feed our children when they depend on us for their nutrition and sustenance will be the food they prefer later.

The increasing amount of time children are spending in front of a screen is having a detrimental effect on their physical, cognitive, and social developments. Computer literacy is important, but recent data are now linking excessive use of the Internet and electronic gadgetry to increases in loneliness and depression, and the implied sedentary activity is associated with obesity and other vascular risk factors. Moreover, playing violent computer games increases aggressiveness and may desensitize the child to pain or suffering in others. For all these reasons, it is recommended that the total amount of time a child spends in front of all screens put together should not exceed two hours per day, and one day a week should be designated as a "No-Screen-Day."

Remember that children learn better and feel happier when there is physical activity in their lives. Encourage them to move and participate as much as you can in their biking, jumping, running, and other workouts. Obesity in preschool children can cause premature and long-term chronic health problems.

It has been associated with academic and social difficulties in kindergarten children, difficulty with social relationships, increased feelings of sadness, loneliness and anxiety, and a negative self-image. These negative consequences of obesity have been noted in children as young as five years of age. In contrast, children who come to enjoy being active will continue to do so as adults. Parents are encouraged to let their children feel the joy of moving their bodies.

In addition to the emphasis on enjoyable physical activity and the avoidance of obesity, the literature is very clear on the positive impact of prolonged exposure to learning and education. The challenge to parents, in addition to infusing their children with the joy of moving their bodies, is to impart to them the love of learning. When the child says, "Why do I need to learn algebra? I will never need it or use it," the answer is "It grows your brain."

Finally, introduce music into the lives of your children early. Musical education and playing an instrument appear to have lasting benefits to cognitive functions, and practising music is well established as a pleasurable means of developing better memory functions.[2] The enjoyment of music, learned at an early age, is a source of lifelong pleasure.

A Message to Health Care Providers

Citizens of all ages entrust their health to their physicians and other health care providers. We shoulder that heavy responsibility, mostly successfully, but it is worth emphasizing a few points in the context of dementia.

1. Hypertension is recognized as the major cerebrovascular risk factor leading to dementia. Please emphasize to your patients that blood pressure must be monitored, and that you expect them to come to their follow-up appointments

ready to share with you their weekly BP values measured at rest.

2. If the resting systolic blood pressure is consistently above 120 mmHg, dietary and lifestyle alterations should be the first approach, but follow-up appointments or calls are crucial to support the patient's resolve to do better. If these conservative measures are insufficient, drug therapy is a must. Orthostatic hypotension with resultant dizziness, falls, and bone fractures are potential consequences of hypertensive therapy, but they are avoidable complications to essential therapy, and patients should be educated on how to avoid them. These potential side effects and complications of hypertensive therapy should not prevent us from protecting the brain.

3. The risk factors for vascular disease and its consequence of dementia are not just rising; they have reached epidemic proportions, and now start at an earlier age. As care providers interested in the long-term health of our patients, we must proactively attempt to correct the lifestyle and vascular risk factors that lead to dementia, starting with the very first years of life.

4. It is important to identify obesity in children under the age of five and intervene, yet less than 50% of us who specialize in pediatric care do so. Obesity in preschool children has been associated not only with health problems but also with poor performance at school. The emotion most often reported to precede an episode of binge eating is anger, highlighting the relationship of food consumption to feelings. Other data show a link between loneliness and the metabolic syndrome. Thus it is important to recognize

and deal with the emotional and social factors that play a role in inducing obesity.

5. A number of common over-the-counter drugs have been linked to a reduction in cognitive function. These include anticholinergic drugs to treat depression, antihistamines for allergies, drugs that treat urinary incontinence, and drugs that help patients fall asleep. The reluctance that many of us now have to prescribing these medications, except in the short term, is appropriate and needs to continue.

6. Please include the caregiver to a person with dementia in your discussions and future planning for the patient. Create a connection with them. Caregivers suffer emotion-ally as they "lose" the affected individual, yet frequently feel compelled to be there for them. They are at great risk for depression and exhaustion. They often need to be nudged by you to take the important step of organizing alternative living arrangements for the affected individual such as placement in a care facility.

7. If you are a health care provider to residents in old age or nursing homes, please resist the temptation to medicalize the residents into submission. Data from some Canadian provinces show that 38% of long-term-care residents are on antipsychotic drugs, frequently prescribed to sedate them. The real goal of this approach is to reduce the care burden on the staff, but it accelerates the decline in the physical and mental abilities of the residents. The only justification for these medications in old age is if the resi-dent poses a threat to self or others.

8. You should take upon yourself, if you are the physician to a long-term-care facility, the responsibility to educate

the staff on the consequences of limiting the residents' mobility. Rather than insisting that wheelchairs be used to move around, programs to enhance the mobility of the residents would directly benefit the individuals and secondarily reduce the care requirements and burden to the staff.

A Message to Educators

The average weight of an American child has risen by more than 11 pounds in the past three decades. A third of the country's children are now overweight or obese. And it's not much different in Canada. Teachers and educators have a particular responsibility in this regard, which they share with the parents. Kids are just not as active as they used to be. With more kids in each class, and fewer resources, physical education programs are often cut first, despite the growing evidence that this hinders student learning.

Some school districts have been assuming a greater responsibility to provide opportunities for the students to exercise, including weaving the activity into the classroom:

1. A DVD called *Brain Breaks* has been developed by Oregon State University. It is a five-minute exercise routine made for classroom use. These breaks were enjoyed by the children, and they also improved their focus, memory functions, and learning ease.

2. Ontario teacher Sheryl Parker sees the results of mini-exercise breaks first-hand in her alternative student program, and she has noted that those who show the most improvement with exercise are students with attention deficit disorders. A day in her class includes music,

cross-crawling, 30-second dance parties, meditation, stretches, and once-a-week runs and problem-solving challenges incorporated into physical games.

3. Educate children and adolescents to take the measures necessary to reduce head injury.

4. School boards and school principals should mandate exercise breaks and monitor them so they do not become opportunities to stand in a corner and rest or text.

5. In high school, later start times may help. Compared to adults, teens prefer to stay up late and sleep later in the morning. Consequently, many teens get far less sleep than they need with early school starts. In response, some school districts have modified the start times for school to later in the morning.

6. There has been a move towards schools selling foods of better nutritional quality, but this laudable trend needs to expand while at the same time reducing the opportunities to circumvent the system by heading over to a fast food joint close by.

A Message to Caregivers of Cognitively Impaired Individuals

The majority of care for patients with dementia is provided at home by family caregivers. Family caregivers often end up being patients themselves, so it is important that caregivers to people with dementia be aware of their own physical and psychological health, and react appropriately.

1. If you are a caregiver to a person who is cognitively impaired, your own health and well-being may be at risk.

If you are a son or a daughter caring for a parent with dementia, you may want to give back to them some of the dedication and love they showed you over the decades, but you should not allow your own health to be undermined.

2. Explore and call upon help that may be available to you through your employer, your municipality, or your health care institution, or through the affected individual's prior professional and social benefits plans, such as with veterans.

3. Express your emotions. Do not isolate yourself. Assuming the mantle of the hero or the poor victim will have negative consequences to your mental health and ability to continue providing care.

4. Call on volunteer organizations to help you. The Alzheimer Society has great educational programs and can provide support if and when needed. Respite facilities can often be accessed through the municipality or, if you can afford it, privately.

5. Music therapy has proven its value. Studies have shown that music therapy for as little as six weeks reduces agitation and disruptiveness in people with dementia. You may be able to apply this and other techniques to reduce the care load on yourself as well as help the affected individual.

6. It is important, perhaps in consultation with others in the family who feel connected with the person with dementia, to define up front the plan of care, keeping in mind that your ability to persevere depends on the intensity and duration of the care needed by the affected person.

7. Remember that up to 38% of family caregivers experience depression, so watch out for it, and react before the feelings of sadness become chronic and debilitating.

8. Setting limits is especially needed if the caregiver is a woman. Research shows that females are at higher risk for assuming an increasing care burden. Also, women care providers seem to get less support from family and society than their male caregiver counterparts.

9. Sooner or later, the decision to institutionalize the individual must be made. You can roughly predict when that step will be unavoidable. Institutionalization will be sooner rather than later if:

   a. The dementia becomes more severe. Lower cognitive and functional abilities and more neuropsychiatric symptoms predict a shorter time until institutionalization.

   b. Bodily functions are not controlled.

   c. Psychiatric symptoms such as agitation, violence, or unpredictable aggression become part of the picture.

If any of these complications become apparent, you should plan on transferring your charge to an institution sooner rather than later.

The Role of Public Policy

In Canada, 8 million Canadians, more than 20% of the population, provide continuing care for relatives or close friends who have long-term health challenges, dementia being prominent among them. This is aggravated by the change in our demographic landscape. By 2030, there will be more people in North America over the age of 60 than under the age of 15, a situation that already exists in Europe. As a result, 1.5 million Americans currently reside in nursing homes where they are often treated more like patients than residents. One of the reasons for this situation is that not only has mortality fallen and longevity is now an accepted reality, but also fertility has fallen. This is creating a demographic deficit that has important implications for our economies and our social structures. Younger people are the major engine of economic activity, and their proportional numbers in society are declining, while older individuals have increased requirements for health care and pension support, which now must extend over decades instead of short years.

Addressing this issue proactively is imperative if we want to preserve our economic health. Governments need to do the following:

1. Promote fertility by financially supporting parental leaves and affordable child care, and put in place tax provisions to diminish the financial burden of childbearing.

2. Put in place immigration policies to promote the infusion of younger demographics into our societies.

3. Allow longer working years and later retirement options for the highly educated and skilled cohorts among the aging segments of the population.

4. Incorporate dementia risk-reduction and management policies into our public health campaigns starting in the teenage years, and develop and promote anti-dementia strategies that focus on reducing risks and promoting brain health.

5. Reduce the effects of vascular disease through public policy. Vascular disease is the underlying cause in many conditions costly to the individual and the public purse, including stroke, myocardial infarction, kidney disease, many lung and eye conditions, and dementia. The health

sector alone cannot solve this problem: it requires coordinated action across all sectors.

6. Invest in research, including running population-level intervention studies, to increase the evidence base on dementia risk reduction.

7. Consider taxation as a tool to combat consumption of extreme high-calorie and other unhealthy foods and beverages, just as it regulates the sale of alcohol and tobacco products, for the purposes of promoting and protecting population health.

8. Provide tax support for respite care for a family caring for a loved one with dementia at home. That will avoid the cost of placement into a care facility and allow a care provider to continue working and contributing to the economy.

9. Consider rewarding those who are physically active by offering financial incentives such as subsidized gym memberships or subsidizing the cost of acquiring desks that allow working while standing.

Changes can be made, and some success is starting to show the path forward. To give but one example, data from the National Health and Nutrition Examination Surveys show that in 2003, 39% of U.S. children ate fast food on any given day, but that dropped to 33% by the time of the 2009 survey.

A major goal for government policy is to postpone frailty and disability, particularly cognitive deficits and dementia, which substantially increase the cost of elder care. Smoking reduction, a success story of public policy, can provide lessons of how to go about it.

A Lesson from Smoking

Public policy has proven it can be successful and effective—the treatment of smoking is an excellent example. There are still 44 million Americans who smoke, but the good news is that 70% of them say they would like to quit. Similarly in Canada the number of smokers now is the lowest it has ever been. This is the result of coordinated public policy that has advertised that smoking kills, has made it uncomfortable or illegal for smokers to do it in many public venues, enforced bans on tobacco marketing, and raised taxes on cigarettes.

Reducing the burden of dementia on the individual and the nation's economy requires a similar integrated public policy approach. The goal is to maximize the likelihood that healthy inputs improve and protect our brains. A national comprehensive public health strategy targeting dementia is needed and was recommended in the recent report on dementia produced by the Standing Senate Committee on Social Affairs, Science and Technology.[3] Not developing such a strategy will be very costly, as some estimates put the cost of caring for dementia by 2040 to nearly $300 billion annually.

The World Health Organization has developed a program that advises health care providers and governments on ways that help in quitting smoking. The same steps can be used as components that increase the chances of any public policy in the field of health to succeed. It is called "Mpower" and for smoking consists of six steps (see Figure 11).

We and our children need to follow the rules promoted in this book, but a rule is not followed just because it is there. As mentioned earlier, it has been reported that when healthy food was offered in school cafeterias, the students just walked over to a fast food joint if there was one close by. Thus, as with smoking, a national strategy is needed to promote those

M is for Monitoring the rate of tobacco use.

P is for Protecting people from second-hand smoke by enacting laws to preserve public access places free of smoke and encouraging individuals to step outside their homes if they do smoke.

O is for Offer, referring to making help available to individual smokers who wish to quit.

W is for Warning about the health hazards of smoking, through ads, pictures on cigarette boxes, and public lectures.

E is for Enforcement. It is not enough to enact laws and designate smoking spots in work places. The rules must be enforced.

R is for Raising taxes. Smoking rates are highest among the poor and the poorly educated, precisely the groups that aggravate their precarious financial standing by spending on this harmful habit. Raising taxes on cigarettes leads to moderation or abandonment of the habit.

FIGURE 11

Mpower for smokers

measures that will minimize the proportion of dementias arising from modifiable risk factors. Such a national strategy would include the following elements:

- ▸ Monitor dementia prevalence to adjust policy accordingly.

- ▸ Mandate, by law, practices that we know decrease the incidence of vascular disease, such as lowering the salt content in processed foods. California is putting warnings on soft drinks and Mexico, France, and several U.S. states are taxing them. Both Canada and the United States will mandate that calorie counts for the foods we consume in restaurants, particularly fast food outlets, be listed visibly.

- ▸ More effective than listing calorie counts is an indication on the label of the activity cost of the item. Thus, converting the calorie content in those soft drinks (250 calories) into what you have to do to burn those calories (you need to walk five miles) has been proven to be more effective in reducing consumption.

▶ Offer national programs, including small subsidies to help those who want to decrease their risk of dementia.

▶ Physician training is necessary to develop the ability to act as advocates and educators on healthy brain aging. The recent exhortation to family physicians to help their patients both avoid obesity and shed pounds is right on the mark.

▶ Governments and cardiovascular and Alzheimer's disease charities should work together to ensure that this message reaches the general public. Together, by purchasing advertising times, we can educate the public on the measures that reduce the risk for dementia and how to incorporate them into our daily lives.

▶ Raise taxes on high-calorie foods. Taxation is a powerful tool to combat the consumption of inexpensive and easily available high-calorie foods. The Cronut meal referred to earlier was a health hazard. Those who consume such foods regularly will cost the taxpayer eventually because their chances of becoming ill are high. Similarly, chocolate-covered bacon should be taxed and made far more expensive by building in the cost of eventual illness.

▶ Consider rewarding individuals who follow the rules in this book. I mentioned that a small reward for those who bring confirmation from their physicians that their vascular risk factors are under control would be very effective in changing behaviour.

▸ Subsidize the cost of blood pressure cuffs.

▸ Many recently designed neighbourhoods are not walk-able, and it is clear that this increases the risk for vascular disease by forcing a sedentary lifestyle and the development of obesity, diabetes, and hypertension. As well, the reduced opportunity to chat with neighbours increases the sense of loneliness and isolation, major contributors to dementia. Condo developers have succeeded in housing large groups of individuals over narrow spaces. Municipalities should demand that health-promoting adjuncts—pleasant walking space, a community garden, minimum sport facilities, and space to socialize in—be included with every condo design submitted.

Reducing dementia in society is an investment, not a cost. There is currently no drug that can halt, slow, or reverse dementia, but there are actions that can significantly delay its onset and reduce its impact. These actions will impose some costs on our treasuries, but the return on investment is high not only through individual function and pleasure, but also by the cost to the public purse. Dementia is now on the agenda of health ministers around the world but much more needs to be done. Governments need to get in front of this impending major social, health, and economic challenge and invest in reducing the impact of dementia. The growing epidemic of dementia will force us to modify our health care priorities. We can do it proactively through planning, or play catch-up after the epidemic is upon us.

REFERENCES

Before the Rules, A Few Facts

1. Alzheimer's Disease International (ADI), London. October 2015. Copyright © Alzheimer's Disease International.

2. Wilson RS, Boyle PA, Yu L, Barnes LL, Schneider JA, Bennett DA. Life-span cognitive activity, neuropathologic burden, and cognitive aging. *Neurology*. 2013;81(4):314–321.

3. Dreary l J, Gow AJ, Taylor MD, Corley J, Brett C, Wilson V, Campbell H, Whalley LJ, Visscher PM, Porteous DJ, Starr JM. The Lothian Birth Cohort 1936: a study to examine influences on cognitive ageing from age 11 to age 70 and beyond. *BMC Geriatr*. 2007;7:28.

4. Ferrucci L. The Baltimore Longitudinal Study of aging (BLSA): a 50-year-long journey and plans for the future. *J Gerontol A Biol Sci Med Sci*. 2008;63(12):1416–1419.

5. Andric M, Hasson U. Global features of functional brain networks change with contextual disorder. *Neuroimage*. 2015 Aug 15;117:103–113.

6. Milner B. The medial temporal-lobe amnesic syndrome. *Psychiatr Clin North Am*. 2005;28(3):599–611, 609.

7. Scoville WB, Milner B. Loss of recent memory after bilateral hippocampal lesions. 1957. *J Neuropsychiatry Clin Neurosci*. 2000;12(1):103–113.

8. Perl TM, Bédard L, Kosatsky T, Hockin J, Todd ECD, Remis RS. An outbreak of toxic encephalopathy caused by eating mussels contaminated with domoic acid. *N Engl J Med*. 1990;322(25):1775–1780.

9. Teitelbaum JS, Zatorre RJ, Carpenter S, Gendron D, Evans AC, Gjedde A, Cashman NR. Neurologic sequelae of domoic acid intoxication due to the ingestion of contaminated mussels. *N Engl J Med*. 1990;322(25):1781–1787.

10. Maeshima S, Osawa A, Yamane F, Shimaguchi H, Ochiai I, Yoshihara T, Uemiya N, Kanazawa R, Ishihara S. Memory impairment caused by cerebral hematoma in the left medial temporal lobe due to ruptured posterior cerebral artery aneurysm. *BMC Neurol*. 2014;14:44.

Rule 1: Grow Your Brain's Capacity for Cognitive Functions

1. Snowdon DA, Greiner LH, Mortimer JA, Riley KP, Greiner PA, Markesbery WR. Brain infarction and the clinical expression of Alzheimer disease. The Nun Study. *JAMA*. 1997;277(10):813–817.

2. Karcski S. Preventing Alzheimer disease with exercise? *Neurology*. 2012;78(17):e110–e112.

3. Wilson RS, Boyle PA, Yu L, Barnes LL, Schneider JA, Bennett DA. Life-span cognitive activity, neuropathologic burden, and cognitive aging. *Neurology*. 2013;81(4):314–321.

4. Kesler S, Hosseini SMH, Heckler C, Janelsins M, Palesh O, Mustian K, Morrow G. Cognitive training for improving executive function in chemotherapy-treated breast cancer survivors. *Clin Breast Cancer*. 2013;13(4):299–306.

5. Griffith-Greene M. Brain training games: no proof they prevent cognitive decline. CBC News Posted: Apr 10, 2015 5:00 AM ET Last Updated: Apr 10, 2015 9:20 AM ET.

6. Gow A, Bastin M, Munoz-Maniega S, Valdes-Hernandez MC, Morris Z, Murray C, Royle N, Starr JM, DearyIJ, Wardlaw JM. Neuroprotective lifestyles and the aging brain, activity, atrophy, and white matter integrity. *Neurology*. 2014;79(17):1802–1808.

7. Harlow JM. "Recovery from the passage of an iron bar through the head." *Publications of the Massachusetts Medical Society*. 1868;2(3): 327–347.

8. Julayanont P, Brousseau M, Chertkow H, Phillips N, Nasreddine ZS. Montreal Cognitive Assessment Memory Index Score (MoCA-MIS) as a predictor of conversion from mild cognitive impairment to Alzheimer's disease. *Dement Geriatr Cogn Disord*. 2006;22:244–249.

9. Sweet L, Van Adel M, Metcalf V, Wright L, Harley A, Leiva R, Taler V. The Montreal Cognitive Assessment (MoCA) in geriatric rehabilitation: psychometric properties and association with rehabilitation outcomes. *Int Psychogeriatr*. 2011;23(10):1582–1591.

Rule 2: Reduce the Debit Calls on Your Mind

1. Lindesay J, Bullock R, Daniels H, Emre M, Förstl H, Frölich L, Gabryelewicz T, Martínez-Lage P, Monsch AU, Tsolaki M, van Laar T. Turning principles into practice in Alzheimer's disease. *Int J Clin Pract*. 2010;64(10):1198–1209.

2. Agüero-Torres H, Kivipelto M, von Strauss E. Rethinking the dementia diagnoses in a population-based study: what is Alzheimer's disease and what is vascular dementia? *Dement Geriatr Cogn Disord*. 2006;22:244–249.

3. Toledo JB, Arnold SE, Raible K, Brettschneider J. Contribution of cerebrovascular disease in autopsy confirmed neurodegenerative disease cases in the National Alzheimer's Coordinating Centre. *Brain*. 2013;136:2697–2706.

4. Kalaria RN, Akinyemi R, Ihara M. Stroke injury, cognitive impairment and vascular dementia. *Biochim Biophys Acta*. 2016;1862(5):915–925.

5. Shih AY, Blinder P, Tsai PS, Friedman B, Stanley G, Lyden PD, Kleinfeld D. The smallest stroke: occlusion of one penetrating vessel leads to infarction and a cognitive deficit. Nat Neurosci. 2013 Jan;16(1):55-63. doi: 10.1038/nn.3278.

6. Papp KV, Kaplan RF, Springate B, Moscufo N, Wakefield DB, Guttmann CR, Wolfson L. Processing speed in normal aging: effects of white matter hyperintensities and hippocampal volume loss. *Neuropsychol Dev Cogn B Aging Neuropsychol Cogn*. 2014;21(2):197–213.

7. Vermeer SE, Longstreth WT Jr, Koudstaal PJ. Silent brain infarcts: a systematic review. *Lancet Neurol.* 2007;6(7):611–619.

8. Weller RO, Yow HY, Preston SD, Mazanti I, Nicoll JA. Cerebrovascular disease is a major factor in the failure of elimination of Abeta from the aging human brain: implications for therapy of Alzheimer's disease. *Ann NY Acad Sci.* 2002;977:162–168.

9. Whitehead SN, Hachinski VC, Cechetto DF. Interaction between a rat model of cerebral ischemia and beta-amyloid toxicity: inflammatory responses. *Stroke.* 2005;36(1):107–112.

10. Iadecola C. The pathobiology of vascular dementia. *Neuron.* 2013;80(4):844–866.

11. O'Donnell MJ, Xavier D, Liu L, Zhang H, Chin SL, Rao-Melacini P, Rangarajan S, Islam S, Pais, McQueen MJ, Mondo C, Damasceno A, Lopez-Jaramillo P, Hankey GJ, Dans AL, Yusoff K, Truelsen T, Diener H-C, Sacco RL, Ryglewicz D, Czlonkowska A, Weimar C, Wang X, Yusuf S, INTERSTROKE INVESTIGATORS. Risk factors for ischaemic and intracerebral haemorrhagic stroke in 22 countries (the INTERSTROKE study): a case-control study. *Lancet.* 2010;376 (9735):112–123.

12. Romàn GC, Nash DT, Fillit H. Translating current knowledge into dementia prevention. *Alzheimer Dis Assoc Disord.* 2012;26(4):295–299.

13. Kivipelto M, Ngandu T,Laatikainen T, Winblad B, Soininen H, Tuomilehto J. Risk score for the prediction of dementia risk in 20 years among middle aged people: a longitudinal, population-based study. Lancet Neurol. 2006;5(9):735-741.

14. Barnes DE, Yaffe K. The projected effect of risk factor reduction on Alzheimer's disease prevalence. *Lancet Neurol.* 2011;10(9):819–828.

15. Bialystok E, Craik FI, Freedman M. Bilingualism as a protection against the onset of symptoms of dementia. *Neuropsychologia.* 2007;45(2):459–464.

16. Perani D, Abutalebi J. Bilingualism, dementia, cognitive and neural reserve. *Curr Opin Neurol.* 2015;28(6):618–625.

17. Van Rooij FG, Schaapsmeerders P, Maaijwee NA, van Duijnhoven DA, de Leeuw FE, Kessels RP, van Dijk EJ. Persistent cognitive impairment after transient ischemic attack. *Stroke.* 2014;45(8):2270–2274.

18. Rajab AS, Crane DE, Middleton LE, Robertson AD, Hampson M, MacIntosh BJ. A single session of exercise increases connectivity in sensorimotor-related brain networks: a resting-state fMRI study in young healthy adults. *Front Hum Neurosci.* 2014;8:625.

19. Tricco AC, Soobiah C, Berliner S, Ho JM, Ng CH, Ashoor HM, Chen MH, Hemmelgarn B, Straus SE. Efficacy and safety of cognitive enhancers for patients with mild cognitive impairment: a systematic review and meta-analysis. *CMAJ.* 2013;185(16):1393–1401.

Rule 3: Monitor and Tame Your Blood Pressure

1. Launer LJ, Masaki K, Petrovitch H, Foley D, Havlik RJ. The association between midlife blood pressure levels and late-life cognitive function. The Honolulu-Asia Aging Study. *JAMA.* 1995;274(23):1846-1851.

2. Muller M, Sigurdsoon S, Kjartansson O, Aspelund T, Lopez OL, Jonnson PV, Harris TB, van Buchem M, Gudnason V, Launer LJ. Age, Gene/Environment Susceptibility-Reykjavik Study Investigators. Joint effect of mid- and late-life blood pressure on the brain: the Ages Reykjavik study. *Neurology.* 2014;82(24):2187–2195.

3. Sugar Intake for adults and children. World Health Organization. http://www.who.int/nutrition/publications/guidelines/sugars_intake/en/.

4. Anstey KJ, von Sanden C, Salim A, O'Kearney R. Smoking as a risk factor for dementia and cognitive decline: a meta-analysis of prospective studies. *Am J Epidemiol.* 2007;166(4):367–378.

5. Neiman J. Alcohol as a risk factor for brain damage: neurologic aspects. *Alcohol Clin Exp Res.* 1998;22(7):346S–351S.

6. Ginty AT, Carroll D, Roseboom TJ, Phillips AC, de Rooij SR. Depression and anxiety are associated with a diagnosis of hypertension 5 years later in a cohort of late middle-aged men and women. *J Hum Hypertens.* 2013;27(3):187–190. doi: 10.1038/jhh.2012.18. Epub 2012 May 17.

7. Wellenius GA, Boyle LD, Coull BA, Milberg WP, Gryparis A, Schwartz J, Mittleman MA, Lipsitz LA. Residential proximity to nearest major roadway and cognitive function in community-dwelling seniors: results from the MOBILIZE Boston Study. *J Am Meriatr Soc.* 2012;60(11):2075–2080.

8. Tonne C, Elbaz A, Beevers S, Singh-Manoux A. Traffic-related air pollution in relation to cognitive function in older adults. *Epidemiology.* 2014;25(5):674–681.

9. Stokholm ZA, Bonde JP, Christensen KL, Hansen AM, Kolstad HA. Occupational noise exposure and the risk of hypertension. *Epidemiology.* 2013;24(1):135–142.

10. Perkovic V, Rodgers A. Redefining Blood-Pressure Targets—SPRINT Starts the Marathon. *N Engl J Med.* 2015;373:2175–2178.

11. Vibo R, Kõrv L, Väli M, Tomson K, Piirsoo E, Schneider S, Kõrv J. Stroke awareness in two Estonian cities: better knowledge in subjects with advanced age and higher education. *Eur Neurol.* 2013;69(2):89–94.

12. Caffrey C, Sengupta M, Park-Lee E, Moss A, Rosenoff E, Harris-Kojetin L. Residents living in residential care facilities: United States, 2010. *NCHS Data Brief.* 2012;(91):1–8.

13. Statistics Canada. High blood pressure, 2012. www.statcan.gc.ca/pub/82-625-x/2013001/article/11839-eng.htm.

14. Leenen FH, Dumais J, McInnis NH, Turton P, Stratychuk L, Nemeth K, Moy Lum-Kwong M, Fodor G. Results of the Ontario survey on the prevalence and control of hypertension. *CMAJ.* 2008;178(11):1441–1449. doi: 10.1503/cmaj.071340.

15. Roberts DF, Foehr UG, Rideout V (Kaiser Family Foundation). Generation M: media in the lives of 8 to 18 year olds. A Kaiser Family Foundation Study. March 2005.

16. Tremblay MS, LeBlanc AG, Kho ME, Saunders TJ, Larouche R, Colley RC, Goldfield G, Connor Gorber S. Systematic review of sedentary behaviour and health indicators in school-aged children and youth. *Int J Behav Nutr Phys Act*. 2011;8:98.

17. Yoon SS, Burt V, Louis T, Carroll MD. Hypertension among adults in the United States, 2009–2010. *NCHS Data Brief*. 2012;(107):1–8.

18. Geleijnse JM, Kok FJ, Grobbee DE. Impact of dietary and lifestyle factors on the prevalence of hypertension in Western populations. *European Journal of Public Health*. 2004;14:235–239.

19. Skoog I, Lithell H, Hansson L, Elmfeldt D, Hofman A, Olofsson B, Trenkwalder P, Zanchetti A, SCOPE Study Group. Effect of baseline cognitive function and antihypertensive treatment on cognitive and cardiovascular outcomes: Study on Cognition and Prognosis in the Elderly (SCOPE). *Am J Hypertens*. 2005;18(8):1052–1059.

20. Skoog I, Andreasson LA, Landahl S, Lernfelt B. A population-based study on blood pressure and brain atrophy in 85-year-olds. *Hypertension*. 1998;32(3):404–409.

21. Peters R, Beckett N, Forette F, Tuomilehto J, Clarke R, Ritchie C, Waldman A, Walton I, Poulter R, Ma S, Comsa M, Burch L, Fletcher A, Bulpitt C, HYVET investigators. Incident dementia and blood pressure lowering in the Hypertension in the Very Elderly Trial cognitive function assessment (HYVET-COG): a double-blind, placebo controlled trial. Lancet Neurol. 2008;7(8):683–689.

22. Vinyoles E, De la Figuera M, Gonzalez-Segura D. Cognitive function and blood pressure control in hypertensive patients over 60 years of age: COGNIPRES study. *Curr Med Res Opin*. 2008;24(12):3331–3339.

23. Jaffe MG, Lee GA, Young JD, Sidney S, Go AS. Improved blood pressure control associated with a large-scale hypertension program. *JAMA*. 2013;310(7):699–705.

24. McAlister FA, Wilkins K, Joffres M, Leenen FH, Fodor G, Gee M, Tremblay MS, Walker R, Johansen H, Campbell N. Changes in the rates of awareness, treatment and control of hypertension in Canada over the past two decades. CMAJ. 2011;183(9):1007-1013.

25. Kaczorowski J, Chambers LW, Dolovich L, Paterson JM, Karwalajtys T, Gierman T, Farrell B, McDonough B, Thabane L, Tu K, Zagorski B, Goeree R, Levitt CA, Hogg W, Laryea S, Carter MA, Cross D, Sabaldt RJ. Improving cardiovascular health at population level: 39 community cluster randomised trial of Cardiovascular Health Awareness Program (CHAP). *BMJ*. 2011;342:d442.

Rule 4: Eat Right, Weigh Light, and Stay Bright!

1. Han TS, van Leer EM, Seidell JC, Lean ME. Waist circumference action levels in the identification of cardiovascular risk factors: prevalence study in a random sample. *BMJ*. 1995;311(7017):1401–1405.

2. Ford ES, Maynard LM, Li C. Trends in mean waist circumference and abdominal obesity among US adults, 1999–2012. *JAMA*. 2014;312(11):1151–1153.

3. Krukowski RA, West DS, Philyaw Perez A, Bursac Z, Phillips MM, Raczynski JM. Overweight children, weight-based teasing and academic performance. *Int J Pediatr Obes*. 2009;4(4):274–280.

4. Mikkilä V, Räsänen L, Raitakari OT, Pietinen P, Viikari J. Consistent dietary patterns identified from childhood to adulthood: the cardiovascular risk in Young Finns Study. *Br J Nutr*. 2005;93(6):923–931.

5. Szalay C, Aradi M, Schwarcz A, Orsi G, Perlaki G, Németh L, Hanna S, Takács G, Szabó I, Bajnok L, Vereczkei A, Dóczi T, Janszky J, Komoly S, Örs Horváth P, Lénárd L, Karadi Z. Gustatory perception alterations in obesity: An fMRI study. *Brain Res*. 2012;1473:131–140.

6. Li W, Prakash R, Chawla D, Du W, Didion SP, Filosa JA, Zhang Q, Brann Dw, Lima VV, Tostes RC, Ergul A. Early effects of high-fat diet on neurovascular function and focal ischemic brain injury. *Am J Physiol Regul Integr Comp Physiol*. 2013;304(11):R1001–1008.

7. Akbaraly TN, Hamer M, Ferrie JE, Lowe G, Batty GD, Hagger-Johnson G, Singh-Manoux A, Shipley MJ, Kivimäki M. Chronic inflammation as a determinant of future aging phenotypes. *CMAJ*. 2013/185(16):E763–770.

8. Wilson PW, D'Agostino RB, Sullivan L, Parise H, Kannel WB. Overweight and obesity as determinants of cardiovascular risk: the Framingham experience. *Arch Intern Med*. 2002;162:1867–1872.

9. Launer LJ, Ross GW, Petrovitch H, Masaki K, Foley D, White LR, Havlik RJ. Midlife blood pressure and dementia: the Honolulu-Asia aging study. *Neurobiol Aging*. 2000;21(1):49–55.

10. Xu WL, Atti AR, Gatz M, Pedersen NL, Johansson B, Fratiglioni L. Midlife overweight and obesity increase late-life dementia risk: a population-based twin study. *Neurology*. 2011;76(18):1568–1574.

11. Schwartz DH, Leonard G, Perron M, Richer L, Syme C, Veillette S, Pausova Z, Paus T. Visceral fat is associated with lower executive functioning in adolescents. *Int J. Obes* (Lond). 2013;37(10):1336–1343.

12. Debette S, Beiser A, Hoffmann U, Decarli C, O'Donnell CJ, Massaro JM, Au R, Himali JJ, Wolf PA, Fox CS, Seshadri S. Visceral fat is associated with lower brain volume in healthy middle-aged adults. *Ann Neurol*. 2010;68(2):136–144.

13. Huang CC, Chung CM, Leu HB, Lin LY, Chiu CC, Hsu CY, Chiang CH, Huang PH, Chen TJ, Lin SJ, Chen JW, Chan WL. Diabetes mellitus and the risk of Alzheimer's disease: a nationwide population-based study. *PLoS One*. 2014;9(1):e87095.

14. Martin AA, Davidson TL. Human cognitive function and the obesogenic environment. *Physiol Behav*. 2014;136:185–193.

15. Kerti L, Witte AV, Winkler A, Grittner U, Rujescu D, Flöel A. Higher glucose levels associated with lower memory and reduced hippocampal microstructure. *Neurology*. 2013;81(2):1746–1752.

16. Alosco ML, Spitznagel MB, Strain G, Devlin M, Cohen R, Paul R, Crosby RD, Mitchell JE, Gunstad J. Improved memory function two years after bariatric surgery. *Obesity* (Silver Spring). 2014;22(1):32–38.

17. National Institutes of Health. Your guide to lowering your blood pressure with DASH. http://www.nhlbi.nih.gov/files/docs/public/heart/new_dash.pdf.

18. Smith PJ, Blumenthal JA, Babyak MA, Craighead L, Welsh-Bohmer KA, Browndyke JN, Strauman T, Sherwood A. Effects of the dietary approaches to stop hypertension diet, exercise, and caloric restriction on neurocognition in overweight adults with high blood pressure. *Hypertension*. 2010;55:1331–1338.

19. Scarmeas N, Stern Y, Mayeux R, Luchsinger JA. Mediterranean diet, Alzheimer disease, and vascular mediation. *Arch Neurol*. 2006;63(12):1709–1717.

20. Esposito K, Maiorino ML, Bellastella G, Chiodini P, Panagiotakos D, Giugliano D. A journey into a Mediterranean diet and type 2 diabetes: a systematic review with meta-analyses. *BMJ Open*. 2015 Aug 10;5(8):e008222.

21. Crous-Bou M, Fung TT, Prescott J, Julin B, Du M, Sun Q, Rexrode KM, Hu FB, De Vivo I. Mediterranean diet and telomere length in Nurses' Health Study: population based cohort study. *BMJ*. 2014 Dec 2;349:g6674.

22. Otto MC, Padhye NS, Bertoni AG, Jacobs DR Jr, Mozaffarian D. Everything in moderation—dietary diversity and quality, central obesity and risk of diabetes. *PLoS One*.2015;10(10):e0141341.

23. Mosconi L, Murray J, Tsui WH, Li Y, Davies M, Williams S, Pirraglia E, Spector N, Osorio RS, Glodzik L, McHugh P, de Leon MJ. Mediterranean diet and magnetic resonance imaging assessed brain atrophy in cognitively normal individuals at risk for Alzheimer's disease. *J Prev Alzheimers Dis*. 2014;1(1):23–32.

24. Tangney CC. DASH and Mediterranean-type dietary patterns to maintain cognitive health. *Curr Nutr Rep*. 2014;3(1):51–61.

25. Bao Y, Han J, Hu FB, Giovannucci EL, Stampfer MJ, Willett WC, Fuchs CS. Association of nut consumption with total and cause-specific mortality. *N Engl J Med*. 2013;369(21):2001–2011.

26. Mattes RD, Kris-Etherton PM, Foster GD. Impact of peanuts and tree nuts on body weight and healthy weight loss in adults. *J Nutr*. 2008;138(9):1741S–1745S.

27. Daniel CR, Cross AJ, Koebnick C, Sinha R. Trends in meat consumption in the United States. *Public Health Nutr*. 2011;14(4):575–583.

28. Chiu CC, Su KP, Cheng TC, Liu HC, Chang CJ, Dewey ME, Stewart R, Huang SY. The effects of omega-3 fatty acids monotherapy in Alzheimer's disease and mild cognitive impairment: a preliminary randomized double-blind placebo-controlled study. *Prog Neuropsychopharmacol Biol Psychiatry*. 2008;32(6):1538–1544.

29. de Souza RJ, Mente A, Maroleanu A, Cozma AI, Ha V, Kishibe T, Uleryk E, Budylowski P, Schünemann H, Beyene J, Anand SS. Intake of saturated and trans unsaturated fatty acids and risk of all cause mortality, cardiovascular disease, and type 2 diabetes: systematic review and meta-analysis of observational studies. *BMJ*. 2015;351:h3978.

30. Grimes CA, Wright JD, Liu K, Nowson CA, Loria CM. Dietary sodium intake is associated with total fluid and sugar-sweetened beverage consumption in US children and adolescents aged 2–18 y: NHANES 2005-2008. *Am J Clin Nutr*. 2013;98(1):189–196.

31. Mathias KC, Slining MM, Popkin BM. Foods and beverages associated with higher intake of sugar-sweetened beverages. *Am J Prev Med*. 2013;44(4):351–357.

32. InterAct Consortium, Romaguera D, Norat T, Wark PA, Vergnaud AC, Schulze MB, van Woudenbergh GJ, Drogan D, Amiano P, Molina-Montes E, Sánchez MJ, Balkau B, Barricarte A, Beulens JW, Clavel-Chapelon F, Crispim SP, Fagherazzi G, Franks PW, Grote VA, Huybrechts I, Kaaks R, Key TJ, Khaw KT, Nilsson P, Overvad K, Palli D, Panico S, Quirós JR, Rolandsson O, Sacerdote C, Sieri S, Slimani N, Spijkerman AM, Tjonneland A, Tormo MJ, Tumino R, van den Berg SW, Wermeling PR, Zamara-Ros R, Feskens EJ, Langenberg C, Sharp SJ, Forouhi NG, Riboli E, Wareham NJ. Consumption of sweet beverages and type 2 diabetes incidence in European adults: results from EPIC-InterAct. *Diabetologia*. 2013;56(7):1520–1530.

33. Singh GM, Micha R, Khatibzadeh S, Lim S, Ezzati M, Mozaffarian D; Global Burden of Diseases Nutrition and Chronic Diseases Expert Group (NutriCoDE). Estimated global, regional, and national disease burdens related to sugar sweetened beverage consumption in 2010. *Circulation*. 2015;132(8):639–666.

34. Pursey KM, Stanwell P, Gearhardt AN, Collins CE, Burrows TL. The prevalence of food addiction as assessed by the Yale Food Addiction Scale: a systematic review. *Nutrients*. 2014;6(10):4552–4590.

35. Ng M, Fleming T, Robinson M, Thomson B, et al. Global, regional, and national prevalence of overweight and obesity in children and adults during 1980–2013: a systematic analysis for the Global Burden of Disease Study 2013. *Lancet*. 2014;384(9945):766–781.

36. Hunter GR, Brock DW, Byrne NM, Chandler-Laney PC, Del Corral P, Gower BA. Exercise training prevents regain of visceral fat for 1 year following weight loss. *Obesity* (Silver Spring). 2010;18(4):690–695.

37. Appel LJ, Clark JM, Yeh HC, Wang NY, Coughlin JW, Daumit G, Miller ER, Dalcin A, Jerome GJ, Geller S, Noronha G, Pozefsky T, Charleston J, Reynolds JB, Durkin N, Rubin RR, Louis TA, Brancati FL. Comparative effectiveness of weight-loss interventions in clinical practice. *N Engl J Med*. 2011;365(21):1959–1968.

38. Deckersbach T, Das SK, Urban LE, Salinardi T, Batra P, Rodman AM, Arulpragasam AR, Dougherty DD, Roberts SB. Pilot randomized trial demonstrating reversal of obesity-related abnormalities in reward system responsivity to food cues with a behavioral intervention. *Nutr Diabetes*. 2014 Sep 1;4:e129.

39. Tal A, Wansink B. Fattening fasting: hungry grocery shoppers buy more calories, not more food. *JAMA Intern Med*. 2013;173(12):1146–1148.

40. An R. Beverage consumption in relation to discretionary food intake and diet quality among US adults, 2003 to 2012. *J Acad Nutr Diet*. 2016;116(1):28–37.

41. Robinson E, Almiron-Roig E, Rutters F, de Graaf C, Forde CG, Tudur Smith C, Nolan SJ, Jebb SA. A systematic review and meta-analysis examining the effect of eating rate on energy intake and hunger. *Am J Clin Nutr*. 2014;100(1):123–151.

Rule 5: Move Your Hind to Save Your Mind

1. James Gallagher. Quarter of adults walk just an hour a week, survey finds. BBC News website. May 6, 2013. http://www.bbc.com/news/health-22401589.

2. James Gallagher. Office workers "too sedentary." BBC News website. March 27, 2015. http://www.bbc.com/news/health-32069698.

3. Donley DA, Fournier SB, Reger BL, DeVallance E, Bonner DE, Olfert IM, Frisbee JC, Chantler PD. Aerobic exercise training reduces arterial stiffness in metabolic syndrome. *J Appl Physiol* (1985). 2014;116(11):1396–1404.

4. Jefferis BJ, Whincup PH, Papacosta O, Wannamethee SG. Protective effect of time spent walking on risk of stroke in older men. *Stroke*. 2014;45(1):194–199.

5. Yarrow JF, White LJ, McCoy SC, Borst SE. Training augments resistance exercise induced elevation of circulating brain derived neurotrophic factor (BDNF). *Neurosci Lett*. 2010 Jul 26;479(2):161–165.

6. Hempstead BL. Brain-derived neurotrophic factor: three ligands, many actions. *Trans Am Clin Climatol Assoc*. 2015;126:9–19.

7. Garza AA, Ha TG, Garcia C, Chen MJ, Russo-Neustadt AA. Exercise, antidepressant treatment, and BDNF mRNA expression in the aging brain. *Pharmacol Biochem Behav*. 2004 Feb;77(2):209–220.

8. Jennings GL, Nelson L, Esler MD, Leonard P, Korner PI. Effects of changes in physical activity on blood pressure and sympathetic tone. *J Hypertens Suppl*. 1984;2(3):S139–141.

9. Singh A, Uijtdewilligen L, Twisk JW, van Mechelen W, Chinapaw MJ. Physical activity and performance at school: a systematic review of the literature including a methodological quality assessment. Arch Pediatr Adolesc Med. 2012;166(1):49-55.

10. Gow AJ, Bastin ME, Muñoz Maniega S, Valdés Hernández MC, Morris Z, Murray C, Royle NA, Starr JM, Deary IJ, Wardlaw JM. Neuroprotective lifestyles and the aging brain: activity, atrophy, and white matter integrity. *Neurology*. 2012;79(17):1802–1808.

11. DeFina LF, Willis BL, Radford NB, Gao A, Leonard D, Haskell WL, Weiner MF, Berry JD. The association between midlife cardiorespiratory fitness levels and later-life dementia: a cohort study. *Ann Intern Med*. 2013;158(3):162–168.

12. Fullston T, Ohlsson Teague EM, Palmer NO, DeBlasio MJ, Mitchell M, Corbett M, Print CG, Owens JA, Lane M. Paternal obesity initiates metabolic disturbances in two generations of mice with incomplete penetrance to the F2 generation and alters the transcriptional profile of testis and sperm microRNA content. *FASEBJ*. 2013;27(10):4226–4243.

13. Naqvi R, Liberman D, Rosenberg J, Alston J, Straus S. Preventing cognitive decline in healthy older adults. *CMAJ.* 2013 Jul 9;185(10):881–885.

14. Chapman SB, Aslan S, Spence JS, Defina LF, Keebler MW, Didehbani N, Lu H. Shorter term aerobic exercise improves brain, cognition, and cardiovascular fitness in aging. *Front Aging Neurosci.* 2013;5:75.

15. Smith JC, Nielson KA, Antuono P, Lyons JA, Hanson RJ, Butts AM, Hantke NC, Verber MD. Semantic memory functional MRI and cognitive function after exercise intervention in mild cognitive impairment. *J Alzheimers Dis.* 2013;37(1):197–215.

16. ten Brinke LF, Bolandzadeh N, Nagamatsu LS, Hsu CL, Davis JC, Miran-Khan K, Liu-Ambrose T. Aerobic exercise increases hippocampal volume in older women with probable mild cognitive impairment: a 6-month randomised controlled trial. *Br J Sports Med.* 2015;49(4):248–254.

17. Williams PT. Lower risk of Alzheimer's disease mortality with exercise, statin, and fruit intake. *J Alzheimers Dis.* 2015;44(4):1121–1129.

18. Liu-Ambrose T, Nagamatsu LS, Graf P, Beattie BL, Ashe MC, Handy TC. Resistance training and executive functions: a 12-month randomized controlled trial. *Arch Intern Med.* 2010;170(2):170–178.

19. de Araújo CC, Silva JD, Samary CS, Guimarães IH, Marques PS, Oliveira GP, do Carmo GRR, Goldenberg RC, Bakker-Abreu I, Diaz BL, Rocha NN, Capelozzi VL, Pelosi P, Rocco PRM. Regular and moderate exercise before experimental sepsis reduces the risk of lung and distal organ injury. *J Appl Physiol.* 2012;112(7):1206–1214.

20. Chudyk A, Petrella RJ. Effects of exercise on cardiovascular risk factors in type 2 diabetes: a meta-analysis. *Diabetes Care.* 2011;34(5):1228–1237.

21. Suchert V, Hanewinkel R, Isensee B. Sedentary behavior and indicators of mental health in school-aged children and adolescents: a systematic review. *Prev Med.* 2015;76:48–57.

22. Simon Whitfield on Outdoor Adventures. Being an Introvert, and His Love Affair with the Stand-Up Paddleboard. http://ahaaliving. com/simonwhitfield. Originally posted February 7, 2015.

23. Bourgomaster KA, Heigenhauser GJ, Gibala MJ. Effect of short-term sprint interval training on human skeletal muscle carbohydrate metabolism during exercise and time trial performance. *J Appl Physiol* (1985). 2006;100(6):2041–2047.

24. Miyashita M, Burns SF, Stensel DJ. Accumulating short bouts of brisk walking reduces postprandial plasma triacylglycerol concentrations and resting blood pressure in healthy young men. *Am J Clin Nutr*. 2008;88(5):1225–1231.

25. Smith PJ, Blumental JA, Babyak MA, Craighead L, Welsh-Bohmer KA, Browndyke JN, Strauman TA, Sherwood A. Effects of the dietary approaches to stop hypertension diet, exercise, and caloric restriction on neurocognition in overweight adults with high blood pressure. *Hypertension*. 2010;55(6):1331–1338.

26. Ngandu T, Lehtisalo J, Solomon A, Levälahti E, Ahtiluoto S, Antikainen R, Bäckman L, Hänninen T, Jula A, Laatikainen T, Lindström J, Mangialasche F, Paajanen T, Pajala S, Peltonen M, Rauramaa R, Stigsdotter-Neely A, Strandberg T, Tuomilehto J, Soininen H, Kivipelto M. A 2 year multidomain intervention of diet, exercise, cognitive training, and vascular risk monitoring versus control to prevent cognitive decline in at-risk elderly people (FINGER): a randomized controlled trial. *Lancet*. 2015;385(9984):2255–2263.

Rule 6: Sleep Enough ... If You Want to Think with Ease!

1. Xie L, Kang H, Xu Q, Chen MJ, Liao Y, Thiyagarajan M, O'Donnell J, Christensen DJ, Nicholson C, Iliff JJ, Takano T, Deane R, Nedergaard M. Sleep drives metabolite clearance from the adult brain. *Science*. 2013;342(6156):373–377.

2. Bellesi M, Pfister-Genskow M, Maret S, Keles S, Tononi G, Cirelli C. Effects of sleep and wake on oligodendrocytes and their precursors. *J Neurosci*. 2013;33(36):14288–14300.

3. Knutson KL. Impact of sleep and sleep loss on glucose homeostasis and appetite regulation. *Sleep Med Clin*. 2007;2(2):187–197.

4. Owens JA, Spirito A, McGuinn M, Nobile C. Sleep habits and sleep disturbance in elementary school-aged children. *Journal of Developmental & Behavioral Pediatrics*. 2000;4(2):67–78.

5. Sexton CE, Storsve AB, Walhovd KB, Johansen-Berg H, Fjell AM. Poor sleep quality is associated with increased cortical atrophy in community-dwelling adults. *Neurology*. 2014;83(11):967–973.

6. Lo JC, Loh KK, Zheng H, Sim SK, Chee MW. Sleep duration and age-related changes in brain structure and cognitive performance. *Sleep*. 2014 Jul 1;37(7):1171–1178.

7. Winsler A, Deutsch A, Vorona RD, Payne PA, Szklo-Coxe M. Sleepless in Fairfax: the difference one more hour of sleep can make for teen hopelessness, suicidal ideation, and substance use. *J Youth Adolesc*. 2015;44(2):362–378.

8. Gamble AL, D'Rozario AL, Bartlett DJ, Williams S, Bin YS, Grunstein RR, Marshall NS. Adolescent sleep patterns and night-time technology use: results of the Australian Broadcasting Corporation's Big Sleep Survey. PLoS One.2014; 9(11): e111700.

9. Lim AS, Kowgier M, Yu L, Buchman AS, Bennett DA. Sleep fragmentation and the risk of incident Alzheimer's sdisease and cognitive decline in older persons. *Sleep*. 2013;36(7):1027–1032.

10. Gelber RP, Redline S, Ross GW, Petrovitch H, Sonnen JA, Zarow C, Uyehara-Lock JH, Masaki KH, Launer LJ, White LR. Associations of brain lesions at autopsy with polysomnography features before death. *Neurology*. 2015;84(3):296–303.

11. Osorio RS, Gumb T, Pirraglia E, Varga AW, Lu SE, Lim J, Wohlleber ME, Ducca EL, Koushyk V, Glodzik L, Mosconi L, Ayappa I, Rapoport DM, de Leon MJ. Sleep disordered breathing advances cognitive decline in the elderly. *Neurology*. 2015;84(19):1964–1971.

12. Guang Y, Lai CSW, Cichon J, Ma L, Li W, Gan W-B. Sleep promotes branch specific formation of dendritic spines after learning. *Science*. 2014;344(6188):1173–1178.

Rule 7: Socialize and Feel Useful: Loneliness and Depression Can Make You Crazy

1. Hawkley LC, Cacioppo J. Loneliness matters: a theoretical and empirical review of consequences and mechanisms. *Ann Behav Med.* 2010;40(2):218–227.

2. Gilmour H. Social participation and the health and well-being of Canadian seniors. *Health Rep.* 2012;23(4):23–32.

3. Vancouver Foundation. Connections and engagement survey. June 2012. http://www.vancouverfoundation.ca/sites/default/files/documents/VanFdn-SurveyResults-Report.pdf.

4. Livingston G. Survey says: we're stressed (and not loving it). *Globe and Mail.* February 2, 2015. http://www.theglobeandmail.com/report-on-business/careers/career-advice/life-at-work/survey-says-were-stressed-and-not-loving-it/article22722102/.

5. Dupre ME, George LK, Liu G, Peterson ED. Association between divorce and risks for acute myocardial infarction. *Circ Cardiovasc Qual Outcomes.* 2015;8(3):244–251.

6. Kross E, Verduyn P, Demiralp E, Park J, Lee DS, Lin N, Shablack H, Jonides J, Ybarra O. Facebook use predicts declines in subjective well-being in young adults. *PLoS One.* 2013;8(8):e69841.

7. Fratiglioni L, Paillard-Borg S, Winblad B. An active and socially integrated lifestyle in late life might protect against dementia. *Lancet Neurol.* 2004;3(6):343–353.

8. Holwerda TJ, Deeg DJ, Beekman AT, van Tilburg TG, Stek ML, Jonker C, Schoevers RA. Feelings of loneliness, but not social isolation, predict dementia onset: results from the Amsterdam Study of the Elderly (AMSTEL). *J Neurol Neurosurg Psychiatry.* 2014;85(2):135–142.

9. Holt-Lunstad J, Smith TB, Layton JB. Social relationships and mortality risk: a meta-analytic review. *PLoS Med.* 2010;7(7):e1000316.

10. Britton A, Shipley MJ. Bored to death? *Int J Epidemiol.* 2010;39(2):370–371.

11. Dufouil C, Pereira E, Chéne G, Glymour MM, Alpérovitch A, Saubusse E, Risse-Fleury M, Heuls B, Salord JC, Brieu MA, Forette F. Older age at retirement is associated with decreased risk of dementia. *Eur J Epidemiol*. 2014;29:253–261.

12. Older workers. US Department of Labor, Bureau of Labor Statistics. July 2008.

13. Living to 109, gerontologist Sister Constance Murphy was a whirlwind of energy. *Globe and Mail*. September 12, 2013.

14. Anderson ND, Damianakis T, Kröger E, Wagner LM, Dawson DR, Binns MA, Bernstein S, Caspi E, Cook SL. The benefits associated with volunteering among seniors: a critical review and recommendations for future research. *Psychol Bull*. 2014;140(6):1505–1533.

15. Renzetti E. Life of solitude: a loneliness crisis is looming. *Globe and Mail*. November 23, 2013. http://www.theglobeandmail. com/life/life-of-solitude-a-loneliness-crisis-is-looming/ article15573187/?page=all.

16. Windle M, Windle R. Recurrent depression, cardiovascular disease, and diabetes among middle-aged and older adult women. *J Affect Disord*. 2013;150(3):895–902.

17. Holt-Lunstad J, Smith TB, Baker M, Harris T, Stephenson D. Loneliness and social isolation as risk factors for mortality: a meta-analytic review. *Perspectives on Psychological Science*. 2015;10(2):227–237.

18. Sclar DA, Robison LM Skaer TL, Galin RS. Ethnicity and the prescribing of antidepressant pharmacotherapy: 1992–1995. *Psychiatry*. 1999;7(1):29–36.

19. Kroenke K, Spitzer R, Williams J. The PHQ-9: validity of a brief depression severity measure. *J Gen Intern Med*. 2001;16:606–613.

20. Bureau of Labor and Statistics. American Time Use Survey: Charts by Topic: Leisure and Sports. www.bls.gov/TUS/CHARTS/LEISURE. HTM.

21. Steffens DC, Welsh-Bohmer KA, Burke JR, Plassman BL, Beyer JL, Gersing KR, Potter GG. Methodology and preliminary results from the neurocognitive outcomes of depression in the elderly study. *J Geriatr Psychiatry Neurol*. 2004;17(4):202–211.

22. Köhler S, van Boxtel MP, van Os J, Thomas AJ, O'Brien JT, Jolles J, Verhey FR, Allardyce J. Depressive symptoms and cognitive decline in community-dwelling older adults. *J Am Geriatr Soc.* 2010;58(5):873–879.

23. Verhoeven JE, van Oppen P, Révész D, Wolkowitz OM, Penninx BW. Depressive and anxiety disorders showing robust, but non-dynamic, 6-year longitudinal association with short leukocyte telomere length. *Am J Psychiatry.* 2016 Mar 4:appiajp201515070887 [Epub ahead of print].

24. Wang L, Leonards CO, Sterzer P, Ebinger M. White matter lesions and depression: a systematic review and meta-analysis. *J Psychiatr Res.* 2014;56:56–64.

25. Aizenstein HJ, Andreescu C, Edelman KL, Cochran JL, Price J, Butters MA, Karp J, Patel M, Reynolds CF 3rd. fMRI correlates of white matter hyperintensities in late-life depression. *Am J Psychiatry.* 2011;168(10):1075–1082.

26. Hakim AM. Depression, strokes and dementia: new biological insights into an unfortunate pathway. *Cardiovasc Psychiatry Neurol.* 2011;2011(2011): Article ID 649629, 6 pages.

27. Sinha R, Lovallo WR, Parsons OA. Cardiovascular differentiation of emotions. *Psychosomatic Medicine.* 1992;54(4):422–435.

28. Wosu AC, Valdimarsdóttir U, Shields AE, Williams DR, Williams MA. Correlates of cortisol in human hair: implications for epidemiologic studies on health effects of chronic stress. *Ann Epidemiol.* 2013;23(12):797–811.

29. Dantzer R, O'Connor JC, Freund GG, Johnson RW, Kelley KW. From inflammation to sickness and depression: when the immune system subjugates the brain. *Nat Rev Neurosci.* 2008;9(1):46–56.

30. Gorelick PB, Counts SE, Nyenhuis D. Vascular cognitive impairment and dementia. *Biochimica et Biophysica Acta.* 1862 (2016) 860–868.

31. Zatorre RJ, Salimpoor VN. From perception to pleasure: music and its neural substrates. *Proc Nati Acad Sci U.S.A.* 2013;110(2):10430–10437.

32. Ripollés P, Rojo N, Grau-Sánchez J, Amengual JL, Càmara E, Marco-Pallarés J, Juncadella M, Vaquero L, Rubio F, Duarte E, Garrido C, Altenmüller E, Münte TF, Rodríguez-Fornells A. Music supported therapy promotes motor plasticity in individuals with chronic stroke. *Brain Imaging Behav*. 2015;pp1–19.

33. Hanna-Pladdy B, Gajewski B. Recent and past musical activity predicts cognitive aging variability: direct comparison with general lifestyle activities. *Front Hum Neurosci*. 2012;6:198.

34. Ericson J. How music strengthens the heart: 30 minutes a day improves cardiovascular function, exercise capacity by 19 percent. *Medical Daily*, Sep 2, 2013.

35. Särkämö T, Tervaniemi M, Laitinen S, Numminen A, Kurki M, Johnson JK, Rantanen P. Cognitive, emotional, and social benefits of regular musical activities in early dementia: randomized controlled study. *Gerontologist*. 2014;54(4):634–650.

36. Hughes CW, Trivedi MH, Cleaver J, Greer TL, Emslie GJ, Kennard B, Dorman S, Bain T, Dubreuil J, Barnes C. DATE: Depressed adolescents treated with exercise: study rationale and design for a pilot study. *Ment Health Phys Act*. 2009;2(2):76–85.

37. Clift S, Hancox G. The significance of choral singing for sustaining psychological wellbeing: findings from a survey of choristers in England, Australia and Germany. *Music Performance Research, Royal Northern College of Music, Special Issue Music and Health*. 2010;3(1):79–96.

38. Evrard AS, Bouaoun L, Champelovier P, Lambert J, Laumon B. Does exposure to aircraft noise increase the mortality from cardiovascular disease in the population living in the vicinity of airports? Results of an ecological study in France. *Noise Health*. 2015;17(78):328–336.

39. Aydin Y, Kaltenbach M. Noise perception, heart rate and blood pressure in relation to aircraft noise in the vicinity of the Frankfurt airport. *Clin Res Cardiol*. 2007;96(6):347–358.

Epilogue

1. Nordstrom P, Nordstrom A, Eriksson M, Wahlund L-O, Gustafson Y. Risk factors in late adolescence for young-onset dementia in men: a nationwide cohort study. *JAMA Intern Med.* 2013;173(17):1612–1618. doi:10.1001/jamainternmed.2013.9079. Published online August 12, 2013.

2. Särkämö T, Tervaniemi M, Laitinen S, Numminen A, Kurki M, Johnson JK, Rantanen P. Cognitive, emotional, and social benefits of regular musical activities in early dementia: randomized controlled study. *Gerontologist.* 2014;54(4):634–650.

3. "Dementia in Canada: A National Strategy for Dementia-friendly Communities." Report of the Standing Senate Committee on Social Affairs, Science and Technology, November 2016.

About the Author

Dr. Hakim obtained his PhD in Biomedical Engineering at Rensselaer Polytechnic Institute in Troy, NY. During his course work for that degree he discovered a real love for medicine, so at the age of 29 he began his medical training at Albany Medical Center in Albany, NY. In 1979 he completed his residency in Neurology at the Montreal Neurological Institute, at which time his career as a neurologist and a brain researcher began. In 1992, Dr. Hakim came to Ottawa to be the University of Ottawa Chair of Neurology and Director of the Neuroscience Research Institute. As well, he was the Division Head of Neurology at the Ottawa Hospital. In 1999, Dr. Hakim initiated the Canadian Stroke Network and was its CEO and Scientific Director during its entire existence from 1999 to 2014. In 2001, he initiated the Heart & Stroke Foundation Centre for Stroke Recovery, and in 2010 he founded the University of Ottawa Brain and Mind Research Institute.

Dr. Hakim's research interests have included the study of stroke and other conditions, the determination of conditions for neuroprotection against ischemic damage, and investigation of post-stroke plasticity and means of enhancing it. During the course of his career, he has published more than 130 scientific papers.

Dr. Hakim is a strong national and international leader in the private, academic, and hospital sectors. He has chaired and served as a member of many committees and boards of granting agencies, foundations, hospitals, and professional associations. In addition to teaching, research, and administrative duties, he maintains clinical functions as a neurologist.

Dr. Hakim has received many honours during his career. In 2007, he was honoured to receive the Thomas Willis Award, a lifetime achievement award from the American Stroke Association. He was appointed Officer of the Order of Canada in 2007. From 2007 to 2012, he was Chair of the European Stroke Network's External Scientific Advisory Committee, Chair of the Best Practice Guidelines Subcommittee of the World Stroke Organization, and a member of that organization's Board of Directors. In 2009, the Heart and Stroke Foundation of Ontario announced an annual research grant to be named the "Dr. Tony Hakim Innovative Stroke Research Award." In January 2011, he received the Hans-Chiari Award, presented to him in Vienna. In June 2012, Dr. Hakim received Her Majesty's Diamond Jubilee Award, and in 2013, he was inducted into the Canadian Medical Hall of Fame.